Lifestyle

The Art of Training Smartly to Burn More Passively, Look Younger and Get Your Ideal Physique

Prateek Asthana

Copyright © 2023 Prateek Asthana
All rights reserved. No part of this publication may be reproduced, distributed or transmitted in any form or by any means including photocopying, recording or other mechanical, electrical methods without the prior written permission of the publisher.

Prateek Asthana is an IT professional by education but by passion; here are some of his key achievements:
- ✓ Certified Fitness Trainer
- ✓ Certified in Sports Nutrition
- ✓ Certified Black Belt Dan-I in Taekwondo (from Orient Combat Arts in association with World Taekwondo Federation, Kukkiwon, Korea)
- ✓ Certified Life Coach
- ✓ Ex-Fitness Consultant in Healthifyme
- ✓ Gold medalist in the Open Taekwondo Corporate Championship held at District Level in Pune under the 66-75Kg Weight Category in 2016
- ✓ Intermediate Level in Boxing & Kickboxing
- ✓ Competed in National and International Half Marathons
- ✓ Certified in First Aid and CPR

and he loves to play outdoor sports like squash, badminton and cricket.

He started his fitness journey around 15 years back with resistance training but hardly knew about nutrition. Prateek has also participated in half marathons from 2015-2018, including one international marathon. He joined martial arts classes in mid-2016 and achieved black belt in 2019 end. In parallel, he also learnt boxing and kickboxing. With years of experience in fitness, he decided to take it to the next level by doing fitness training and sports nutrition certifications, after which he worked as a fitness consultant at HealthifyMe for a short duration.

He respects his primary job and loves learning new things in the fitness industry. Prateek has still not stepped into the world of content creation in social media and does not have a professional account currently, but who knows, we might see him in that world sooner or later if he feels so.
He stays in Pune (India) and will probably be seen in one of the calisthenics classes soon.

You can connect with him on his personal account:
Instagram (prateek_asthana_)
Facebook (www.facebook.com/prateek.asthana.3)

CONTENTS

Why should I go for this content?........................6

Chapter 1: Know Your 'Why': Your 'Why' Must Be > Your Excuses..9

Chapter 2: Don't Rush: It's About Changing Your Habits Eventually..13

Chapter 3: Conventional & Modern Approach to Track Body Composition 16

Chapter 4: How to Know Your Daily Calorie Consumption?..20

Chapter 5: Individual Goal........................22

    Goal – Fat Loss..22

    Goal – Muscle Gain or Hypertrophy 26

    Goal – Maintenance 30

Workout: Key Ingredient to Stay Fit 33

Chapter 6: Training Regimen 33

Chapter 7: Flexibility and Mobility 39

Chapter 8: Good Body Posture and Self-Check.......42

Chapter 9: Cardiovascular Training.........47

Chapter 10: Resistance Training 53

Chapter 11: Muscle Contractions & ATP-ADP Cycle 60

Chapter 12: Training Techniques and Principles ...63

Chapter 13: Strength Workouts for Major Muscle Groups 78

Chapter 14: How to Prepare Your Workout Plan?: Gym & Home Workout 82

Chapter 15: Periodization 103

Chapter 16: How to Measure Your Progress? 106

Chapter 17: Are Supplements Necessary? 108

Chapter 18: Pre, Intra and Post-Workout Intake . 123

Chapter 19: Myths & Facts 126

Chapter 20: Closure 134

Why should I go for this content?

We all want to enjoy the meals and beverages we love and stay fit as well, isn't it?
You don't need to be completely deprived of your favourite meal to get an ideal body shape. Have you ever tried any such diet that demands you to altogether leave certain things you love to lose fat or gain muscles? How long were you able to follow that diet?
Humans don't love restrictions. We will not discuss anything in this book series that completely restricts you from leaving something that you love to have or even forcefully asks you to have anything you don't like.

How is it possible?
You need to understand the process of training smartly and cheating wisely in nutrition as per your goal. To understand the complete process, you must know about the nutrition you must intake as per your goal, along with some physical activity.
This knowledge will make you independent in choosing the nutrition and training plans as per your likes and dislikes and will also help you achieve your ideal body shape regardless of gender.
Everything that we will be discussing in this course is in layman's language and applies to all the age groups of teens and above for any gender. We just need to stay together till the end of the course to understand the basics so that we can apply them in our lifestyle to burn

more calories passively, even in the resting state.

What is this book all about?
This book will completely talk about how to add fitness to our routine. So, suppose you are a beginner or someone struggling to kick-start your journey or keep up the momentum after training for a while. In that case, the book will help you get direction since you will now have the knowledge and know how to train smartly to achieve your specific goal to get an ideal physique. You don't need to listen to everybody and land in confusion. The science behind fitness, the training principles and techniques will help you design and update your workout plans.

Have you already tried everything?
If you feel that you have tried everything before and still failed to keep up your motivation, this is your chance to understand why you have been failing till now.
If you feel that you do everything to lose weight but still don't get results, or you eat healthy food but still fail to get an ideal shape because you don't have a good metabolism or your genes don't support you, can thank me later for sharing all this knowledge and opening your eyes.

An active and healthy lifestyle is not about blindly following someone or something. It is just like the stock market. If you know the fundamentals and technicals of studying stocks, you know where you are investing your hard-earned money, so the basic knowledge of training and nutrition always helps you understand your body.

Do weekend parties don't allow you to progress?
You do everything right, but as the weekend arrives, you love to party and have junk food and drinks, and you return to square one. Don't worry; that's a common problem, so we will also discuss the hack for partying in the upcoming book of the same series, where you will learn to cheat wisely and have drinks and food without creating much disturbance in your goal so that you eventually progress.

Let's get started!
Does it hurt you to count the amount you have invested so far in gym memberships, supplements, or diets without getting any results? In that case, you must thoroughly go through the entire course to apply it to yourself, and this will be the best return on investment that you will ever make in this entire life!
So, let's start with the course, and the first book of a two-book series will talk about fitness and training.

Chapter 1: Know Your 'Why': Your 'Why' Must Be > Your Excuses

Before you understand the process and start your fitness journey, you must be very clear about why you want to start it. This may sound like a fundamental question, but if you have been failing till now and you want to add fitness to your lifestyle, your 'why' must be greater than your excuses. You cannot be motivated every day; you need to be disciplined.

If your goal is to look slim in your wedding dress or any family function, it's good that you have the motivation to start, but it's not good enough to stay in the game for long.

"Fitness is a journey, not a destination; you must continue for the rest of your life." — Kenneth H. Cooper.

Don't treat fitness as a sprint, aligning it with your short-term goals and using unsustainable methods that could have repercussions. It is a life-long marathon, and if you commit to participate, your body will reflect your lifestyle. Don't chase six-pack abs or perfect figures initially; these are all by-products of your dedication and discipline towards a healthy and active lifestyle, which will eventually be achieved if you follow the process.

The beginning is always challenging, but once you adopt a healthy lifestyle, you get addicted to it. Do you remember yourself or anyone else feeling sad or regretting after a good workout session?
This is because a workout session releases endorphins, which help alleviate pain, reduce stress & anxiety, boost self-esteem, and improve overall well-being.

We all deal with different situations throughout our lives that sometimes add stress and ultimately disturb cortisol (stress-regulating hormone) levels, which promotes symptoms like digestive problems, headaches, low sex drive, menstrual problems, high blood sugar levels, and high blood pressure, and the list is quite long.

A healthy lifestyle, including workout and balanced nutrition, keeps you physically and mentally fit. You are mentally and physically more active, leading a better personal and professional life.

As a child, I always remember my father saying, "Either you enjoy the food you love throughout your life, maintaining a healthy lifestyle, or you enjoy it without any limits until you reach a medical condition and the doctor asks you to avoid it". This was my 'why' as a child.

Exercise helps prevent several medical conditions and partially or completely treat certain conditions. It helps to:
- Control certain allergies
- Fight anxiety and depression
- Prevent or treat arthritis
- Reduce back pain problems
- Prevent the development of cancer cells
- Prevent cardiovascular problems
- Prevent and treat digestive problems
- Control cholesterol levels
- Prevent and control diabetes
- Prevent and control blood pressure problems
- Control hormonal imbalances and aids in menstrual problems and PMS
- Prevent and control thyroid problems and PCOS/PCOD
- Prevent lung and kidney problems
- Improve cognitive ability
- Maintain ideal body weight composition
- Maintain bone health
- Boost immunity
- Increase strength
- Increase flexibility

And a lot more. In short, exercise helps to prevent or reduce the probability of one facing a medical condition at an early or later stage of life.

Although these are strong reasons to add fitness into the lifestyle, if these reasons are also not strong enough for you, find out your reason, which is strong enough to stay in the game forever.

Reference - Page 7: Fitness quote from Cooper Cooper Fitness Center Membership Options.
https://www.cooperaerobics.com/Cooper-Fitness-Center-Dallas/General-Information.aspx

Chapter 2: Don't Rush: It's About Changing Your Habits Eventually

Think about changing your habits to kickstart your journey. If you are a novice in this area, start with sparing 30-45 minutes for yourself when you can workout for 4-5 days a week. If you don't have time, you must find time if health is your priority.

If you have access to workout equipment or you can afford to go to the gym, that's great, and we will discuss the details as we progress with the chapters, but if you do not have access to a gym, sports club, or any equipment at the beginning, simply start with walking. Take stairs instead of escalators if you don't have any medical condition that restricts you from doing it.

The idea is to progress gradually, so if you were already walking 5000 steps in your daily routine, increase it to 8000-10000 steps per day eventually, or add any active outdoor sport (badminton, basketball, boxing, cricket, squash, etc.) along with some body weight workouts like squats, push-ups (or knee- assisted push-ups or wall push-ups for beginners) to gain some strength.

You need to take the first step towards your journey, no matter how small it is. If you can spare 30 minutes for yourself to workout regularly, it is a massive step, as most people are not motivated to find time to prioritize their health.

Check your water consumption if it is less. You should drink at least 30ml of water per kilogram of your body weight. Simply divide your weight in kilograms by 30.

If your weight is 60 kg, 60/30 = 2 litres is the bare minimum requirement. Rest depends on factors like the kind of food intake, physical activities, how much you sweat, etc.

Try to sleep for 7-8 hours per day at a stretch and at a fixed time.

If you consume processed food or desserts four times a week, narrow the frequency to 2 times weekly. If you crave fast food or packaged food on most days and bring down the counter directly from 4 to 0, you might get more cravings after some time and lose momentum if you don't see the results, and most beginners measure the progress only on the scale. We will discuss how to measure your actual progress and keep it going.

So, take baby steps for now while you are reading this. Start your journey, and by the end of the book, you will get more knowledge and reasons to add fitness to your lifestyle.

You will get results if you are taking care of workout, nutrition, hydration and recovery. We will discuss them in detail as we move ahead. Initially, we need to give a little push to change our habits, and gradually, your habits will push you back once it is in your routine. You need to be in a relationship with your body, and your body reciprocates the love and care in the form of your fitness level and physique.

Chapter 3: Conventional & Modern Approach to Track Body Composition

BMI

BMI, or Body Mass Index, is a conventional method that categorizes an adult into underweight, normal, overweight, or obese categories per body weight and height.

BMI	Weight Status
Below 18.5	Underweight
18.5 – 24.9	Normal
25 – 29.9	Overweight
30 – 34.9	Obesity, Class I
35 – 39.9	Obesity, Class II
Above 40	Extreme Obesity, Class III

BMI = Weight (Kgs)/Height (m^2)

BMI doesn't account for the ratio of muscle mass and fat mass, which means that a 74 kg person with good muscle mass and 10% body fat having a six-pack falls under the overweight category as per BMI. Although, he might not need to lose any pounds because the extra pounds are of muscle mass.

Hence, it would help if you focused more on BMR while checking body composition involving muscle mass and fat mass percentage rather than focusing on BMI.

BMR

The human body mainly comprises muscle, fat, bone, and fluid. When people say they want to lose weight, they want to lose fat. Unfortunately, the lack of awareness, improper ways of training and FAD diets make them lose muscle mass, which directly hits their metabolism.

The more muscle mass in your body, the more your BMR (Basal Metabolic Rate).
The human body burns calories even in a resting state through essential life-sustaining functions like cell production, breathing, nutrient processing, blood circulation, etc. This is called the Basal Metabolic Rate (BMR).

To calculate your BMR approximately, you can use the Harris-Benedict formula, which considers sex, weight, height, and age.

Cis Female:
BMR = 655.1 + (9.56 * weight in kg) + (1.85 * height in cm) − (4.68 * age in years)

Cis Male:
BMR = 66.5 + (13.75 * weight in kg) + (5 * height in cm) − (6.75 * age in years)

Come on, pick a calculator! Don't be too lazy to calculate even if you hate equations! You don't have to do this every day and this will give you an approximate idea about your BMR!

Your metabolism or BMR decreases with age, and you tend to lose muscle.
Also, one pound of muscle mass is less dense and burns more calories than fat mass, so resistance training and proper nutrition help you gain or maintain muscle mass, and you burn more calories even in a resting state.

Body Composition
Knowing your body composition is more relevant than checking your weight on the scale. Body composition tells you about your muscle mass, fat mass, water mass, bone mass, BMR, metabolic age, and other factors.

You drink one litre of water and measure your weight on a standard weighing scale. What do you think you have gained? Most people still get worried about checking that increment of 1kg, which is your increase in water weight.

Although there are many ways for body composition tests like hydrostatic weighing, bodpod, skinfold callipers, dual-energy x-ray absorptiometry, etc.. I suggest you go for bioelectrical impedance analysis used in gyms or the small devices that come with a weighing scale that needs to be connected through Bluetooth with our cellphone app for that device.

Bioelectrical impedance is the method of passing an electric current (very low) through our body—the current flows quickly when the body has less fat content, higher water, and salts. On the contrary, a body with higher fat mass resists current, and impedance is high.

This method is not very accurate and might have some variance, but it is easily available, portable and reasonable. You can either buy it online or access it in gyms.
You will get a fair idea of your muscle mass, fat mass and other relevant factors using this device, and you can track your progress regularly.

Chapter 4: How to Know Your Daily Calorie Consumption?

Apart from BMR, there are two more terms, 'TDEE' and 'Thermic Effect of Food' which determine your calorie intake, but in the beginning, I don't want you to complicate it. So, I am just giving a brief idea of what they are, but we will keep our formula simple to know the estimated number of calories we need daily.

TDEE (Total Daily Energy Expenditure)
Total Daily Energy Expenditure (TDEE) is the approximate number of calories you burn per day when exercise is considered.

Total Daily Energy Expenditure = Basal Metabolic Rate + Physical Activity + Thermic Effect of Food

Apart from the above formula, TDEE is also calculated by multiplying an activity multiplier by your BMR as per your activity level. You will find an online TDEE calculator on the internet.

Thermic effect of food
The thermic effect of food (specific dynamic action) is an increase in metabolic rate that occurs after consuming a food item. It is the amount of energy required by the body to process, digest and use food. It is estimated around 10% of food energy intake, but this can vary depending on what we are consuming, protein has a far more significant thermic effect

than dietary fat, since it is more difficult to process it.

If you don't have any hormonal imbalance, weight loss (not fat loss) is simple arithmetic:

Weight Loss:
Number of Calories Burnt > Number of Calories Consumed

Weight Gain:
Number of Calories Burnt < Number of Calories Consumed

Maintenance:
Number of Calories Burnt = Number of Calories Consumed

Fact
3500 Kcal = 1 Lb of weight
7700 Kcal = 1 Kg of weight
Don't get confused between calories and Kilocalories. Our daily need is in Kcal and the nutritional value mentioned behind food items are also in Kcal. To simplify things, Kcal is mentioned as Calories ('C' in upper case).

Chapter 5: Individual Goal

Goal – Fat Loss

1. **Be On a Calorie Deficit Diet.**

You must be on a calorie-deficit diet if your goal is to lose fat. I suggest going slow (maximum 500 Cal/day deficit) so that you neither overtrain nor let your body be nutrition-deprived by creating too much deficit.

Since you have already calculated your BMR by now. Keep the formula simple:
Consider your daily burns = BMR + Daily workout (ignoring the ~10% thermal effect of food for now)
If Daily burns – Calories consumed = ~400-500 Calories,
then you will lose approximately one pound (1 pound ~ 3500 Cal) in 7 workout days.
In actuality, if you are losing more than a pound in a week, even after your theoretical calculation is correct, your burns are more, so you can reduce some activity level if you are feeling a little low on energy or you can consume a little more food to reduce the rate of burns/week slightly. It's not a race; you shouldn't burn out or create mineral or vitamin deficiencies while achieving this goal. Keep it slow and steady and we will cover the details of nutrition in the second book of this series.

The number of calories burnt during a daily workout depends on your activity. Your calorie burns depend on your heart rate, which should be 55-85% of your maximum heart rate during a workout session.

Maximum heart rate = 220 – Your Age (in years)

As compared to a cardiovascular session, you burn comparatively fewer calories during a resistance training session, but you still burn calories after a weight training session or HIIT (High-Intensity Interval Training) session because there is an elevation in oxygen consumption and metabolism, which occurs post workout as the body recovers, repairs, and returns to its pre-exercise state. This can occur for up to 24 hours. This state is also called as EPOC (Excess Post-exercise Oxygen Consumption).
As per some studies, EPOC can add 5 to 15 per cent of the total energy cost of the exercise session.

To get a fair idea, if you don't have a smartwatch to track activity, you may burn ~250-300 Calories in a moderate-intensity resistance training session of 45-60 minutes and additional burns of 5-15%, including EPOC.

2. **Which training works best for fat loss?**
Resistance training, along with cardiovascular training, works best for fat loss.
Cardiovascular training helps you lose overall weight (water mass, muscle mass and fat mass), and since losing muscle mass means

degrading your metabolism, you must add resistance training along with cardio.

3. **Walk after the meals.**
It is a great idea to include 15-20 minutes' walk post lunch, dinner or your meals.
Low physical activity like walking post meals has a protective effect your gastrointestinal (GI) tract. It can help in digestion by promoting stimulation of the stomach and intestines, causing food items to move through more quickly.

Walking after eating might also help prevent constipation, ulcers, irritable bowel syndrome, colorectal cancer and heartburn. It may also manage blood sugar levels.
Adding walk post meals can reduce systolic blood pressure by 10%.

4. **Don't go for FAD diets.**
FAD diets are diets known to be a quick fix for obesity. They claim to have faster results but are unsustainable for the long term and do not focus on changing your lifestyle, defying basic principles of nutritional adequacy.

Faster results in health and higher returns in investing always seem attractive to people, isn't it? But, with high return comes high risk, be it wealth or health. So, always focus on the process; you will get results as a by-product.

5. **Don't eat less than your BMR.**

Many people skip meals and eat less for some time to achieve faster results. Nutrition is the fuel for your body. Being on a calorie-deficit diet by just eating less and no physical activity will degrade your metabolism with time since you will initially lose overall weight just for some time to gain fat later when you start consuming your previous maintenance calories.

You need to add physical activity, have balanced nutrition at least equivalent to your BMR or more and then create a deficit to avoid becoming vitamin and minerals deficient with time, which could lead to low energy levels and other side effects negatively impacting your health despite you trying to make efforts to lose some pounds.

6. **Do cardio after your strength training session.**

Start your session with 5-7 minutes of warm-up activities, but perform cardiovascular activities after your strength training session, as it will fatigue your muscles. Use your strength for resistance training to lift more, which helps you build muscle mass and then go for cardiovascular activities at the end of your session. Your glycogen stores will be depleted after your weight training session, and then your body will start breaking down fatty acids if you do a cardio session at the end.

7. **Don't overcompensate.**

If you had a party over the weekend or you had too many calories during a wedding or farewell event, don't try to overcompensate by being on a very low-calorie diet for the next 2-3 days. Too much calorie variation frequently could lead to problems like metabolic abnormalities, hormonal imbalances, menstrual dysfunction, etc.

Just get back to your routine on the next day, do your workout and have proper meals like you were having before your weekend getaway.

8. **Don't go for shortcuts like drinks or belts claiming fat loss.**

There is no shortcut to a healthy and active lifestyle. Food or beverages contain calories. There could be a few beverages that contain very low to almost zero calories, like black coffee, black or green tea, but consuming zero to no calories does not make you lose fat. Only a calorie-deficit diet makes you lose fat.

Yes, replacing morning cold coffee with iced americano (although it might not satisfy your taste buds) would create a difference in your daily calorie consumption. Changing such habits would certainly create a difference. Still, drinking green tea after morning cold coffee will not do the magic.

So is the case with belts or any such product claiming fat loss. Workout with a balanced diet is the key.

Goal – Muscle Gain or Hypertrophy

1. **Be On a Calorie Surplus Diet.**

You must be on a calorie-surplus diet for muscle gain. So, if you consume 3000 Calories and your total daily energy expenditure is 2500 Calories, you will gain one pound in a week ((3000-2500) *7 = 3500 Calories equivalent to one pound).

That is why measuring and tracking food items initially is important if you want to understand the science behind this. Once you get an idea of the quantity of the food items you consume and start understanding your body, you might not need it if you don't like to track.

Do not eat anything just to create a surplus. Your macronutrients ratio should be maintained, or else you might gain more fat mass than muscle mass.

2. **Progressive Overload**

The same workout routine using the same weights, the number of sets and reps leads to a plateau and no more challenges to your muscle fiber. Progressive overload is the increase in the volume of your workout to challenge your muscles to grow muscle size by adding more tension.

You need to achieve this gradually as the strength increases. Balanced nutrition with a calorie-surplus diet gives more fuel to the body, and by progressive overload, you can grow your muscle size with time. Go slow and try to increase the volume in 2 weeks or so as your body allows.

Volume depends on the following factors:
- Add Resistance – If you are lifting a dumbbell of 10kg on a bicep curl, try increasing it to 12.5kg.

- More Repetitions – If you were lifting a 10kg dumbbell on a bicep curl and doing 8 reps, try increasing reps to 9 or 10.
- Increase duration of the workouts – Adding one more set of existing workouts or adding another workout would increase the length of the workout.
- More tempo – Reduce rest between sets to increase tempo.

Doing any one or more of the above would increase your volume of the workout.

Example:
Current scenario
You do 3 sets with 8 reps each of bench press with 40kg weight, and your rest period is 1 minute between sets. (Volume: 3 * 8 * 40 = 960)

After 2 weeks
Increasing weight from 40 to 45kg will increase your volume if other factors are constant.
Increasing reps from 8 to 9 will increase your volume if other factors are constant.
Increasing sets from 3 to 4 will increase your volume if other factors are constant. (No matter if you can do a lesser number of reps in the last set.)
Reducing rest time from 1 minute to 45 seconds, keeping other factors constant.
Increasing weight from 40 to 45, but your reps are reduced to 7, keeping sets and rest time constant, your volume is 3 * 7 * 45 = 945. Although this is less than your initial volume,

that's absolutely fine, and you can push yourself for 8 reps next week.

While picking 45 instead of 40, you would not know if your failure would arrive after 6, 7 or 8 reps, but it still counts as progress. You can also do a mix and match of 3 sets with (45 * 7 reps + 40 * 9 reps + 40 * 8 reps = 995)

3. **Recovery and Rest Between the Muscle Groups Workout.**

Recovery avoids burnout, and it is important for your muscle growth. You must give 48 hours of rest to the muscle group after training. Plan your muscle group workouts accordingly. Workout creates microscopic tears in your muscle tissue, which are repaired during rest. Sleep for 7-8 hours per day. If your schedule allows a quick nap of 15-30 minutes during the daytime and your body needs it, it sometimes aids in recovery and increases performance in the gym. Your rest day is ideally a growth day for muscles. Obviously, that doesn't mean you rest more than you workout :-).

4. **Compound Movement**

Exercises that work more than one muscle group at the same time are compound movements.

For example, bench press is a compound movement that works your chest, shoulders and arms muscles. Similarly, pull-ups and push-ups are also compound movements. On the other hand, preacher curl is an example of isolation movement that targets one main muscle joint.

Compound movements improve intramuscular coordination, flexibility, and strength and help you gain more muscle mass.

For muscle building, try to hit one muscle group twice a week. Compound movements like deadlifts, squats, and bench press help you achieve this.
So, even if you are training for one muscle group each day, like if you are training chest one day, your shoulders and arms are being worked out by compound movements, and your biceps are being worked out with your back workouts.

Goal – Maintenance

1. **Know Your Maintenance Calories and balance your macronutrient ratio**.

If you want to maintain your weight but still feel that your body needs to be in the perfect shape you want to see, it means that your muscle mass and fat mass ratio are not in the ideal proportion. In this scenario, you need to consume calories at par with total daily energy expenditure, but you need to ensure that your macronutrient ratio is maintained while doing resistance training and cardio training, which we discussed above so that you gradually gain muscle mass and lose fat mass.
Apart from having maintenance calories, all other points discussed in the other two goals can also be applied to maintenance.

2. Be a Better Version of Yourself

If you feel that your body is in the ideal shape, that's great, and I am sure you must have worked hard to achieve this phase and will continue this journey, no matter if you have reached the ideal state. I hope you have a new goal in mind, be it to gain more strength, power, flexibility, agility, endurance, etc. Workout as per your goals. With time, you can always learn and work to see a better version of yourself.

Common to Each Goal

Don't Overtrain

Whatever your goal is, do not over-train. Your body needs rest, and you must listen to your body. As a beginner, you should give at least one day of rest per week, and if your body or goal demands 2-3 days of rest, it is perfectly fine.

Overtraining can lead to strain, injuries, fatigue, and weight loss, including muscle mass drop, reduced performance, and disturbed sleep. It can also affect your stress hormone levels.

4-6 days of workout (as per your goal), along with balanced nutrition in your diet, would help you achieve your goals.

With time and experience, you might not feel like resting even after 6-7 days of workout. In that case, take complete or active rest whenever your body demands, and it's completely fine to workout on other days.

Unlike passive rest, where you completely give rest to your body, active rest gives time for your muscles to recover. Meanwhile, you also burn some calories with activities like walking, yoga, stretching or cycling, but avoid leading yourself to exhaustion.

Hydration
Again, no matter what your goal is, be it fat loss or muscle gain or maintenance, hydration is important. You sweat during workouts and lose water and electrolytes. Your sweat contains 99% water and 1% electrolytes. Considering your minimum hydration needs as per your body weight (Weight in kg/30), consume 1 litre or extra daily if you are sweating more. You must also replace the lost electrolytes, so don't compensate it with just water. Water is important, but our human body has a ratio of water and electrolytes that must be maintained. So, you must consume food items or beverages that include sodium, potassium, calcium, magnesium and other minerals to compensate for the loss.

Remember that you also get water from milk, pulses, gravy items in your meals, coffee, tea, juices, etc. So, suppose you are actively consuming 3 litres of water every day, depending on the food and drink items you are having. In that case, you are additionally consuming 0.5-1 or more litres of water daily, which is good.

Workout: Key Ingredient to Stay Fit

Chapter 6: Training Regimen

Training for individuals could differ based on what you are training for. A professional marathon runner's training schedule would vary from a sprinter, boxer or powerlifter.
If you are not training for a professional sport and are a beginner who wants to train because you want to lead an active and healthy lifestyle throughout your life, it is great that you have taken your first step towards this beautiful journey.

In general, a training regimen must include:
- Warm Up
- Main Workout
- Post Workout Stretches

Warm Up
You must warm your body for 5-10 minutes before starting the main workout. Warm-up elevates your heart rate from its resting state and has benefits like:
- More blood flow and oxygen
- Increases flexibility and range of motion
- Lowers injury risk
- Better performance

You can include 3-5 minutes of treadmill jog, cycling or jump rope in your warm-up schedule, and you can also include exercises like jumping jacks and high knee. Such cardio warm-ups elevate your heart rate and increase blood flow post which, depending upon the muscle group you are training for the day, you can include some **dynamic stretches** and **mobility workouts** that help to strengthen your muscles around the joints. Some of the basic warm-up exercises include:

- Upper body: neck rotation, arm rotation, arm crossovers, spinal rotation, wrist sways.
- Lower body: High knees, hip circles, leg swings, squats, walking lunges, lateral lunges, butt kicks, hula hip swings, butterfly movement.

Do the same warm-up exercises apply to everyone?

Warm-up cannot be the same for everyone. People who are into intermediate or advanced training might not feel their muscles getting warmed up by doing the same activities we discussed above for beginners. So, they can include 2 sets of lightweight compound movement workouts after some cardio and dynamic stretches.

Push-ups, pull-ups, lat pull down, bench press with light weights or empty barbell rod. As you progress, you might also have to change the warm-up routine to avoid injuries.

If you reside in an area where the temperature is relatively low, you should spend a little more time getting your body warmed up to start the main workout.

Do not include static stretches in your warm-up schedule. We will discuss them in the post-workout stretches section.

By directly jumping to the main workouts, you will not only put more strain on your heart to pump blood, but you can also invite sprained muscles and injuries.

Main Workout
The main workout would differ for people depending on their goals and the sport they are in.
A professional boxer, powerlifter, cricketer, football, tennis player, or marathon runner will have different workout plans, but the one thing in common is resistance training. They need to have the strength to improve their performance in sports.

If you are not into professional training, you can choose from different activities as per your interest. You can go for yoga, calisthenics, martial arts, sports, weight training, zumba, functional training or any other activity.
The important thing you need to remember is that if your activity involves only cardiovascular training, you will lose weight. Still, you will ultimately lose muscle mass and degrade your metabolism (BMR), which we

discussed earlier. So, your workout routine must include any resistance training, if not on all days, at least on alternate days, to gain muscle strength and improve metabolism.

In short, cardiovascular exercises are good if your vision is to stay slim with a healthy heart. However, if you wish to have an appealing physique and ideal body composition, be it leaner, you must strengthen your muscles. Your workout plan must have resistance training if you want to get an ideal body shape!

We will discuss cardiovascular and resistance training in detail in the upcoming chapters.

Post Workout Stretches
You must do static stretches as a part of post-workout stretches. These stretches demand muscles to stretch beyond a point, and one is supposed to hold the position for 10-30 seconds to help loosen and lengthen your muscles and connective tissue. Since you are stretching your muscles to a point of very mild discomfort, your body should already be warmed up. You should not include static stretches in warm-ups to avoid injuries and negative performance impacts.

When you push through an intense workout, lactic acid accumulates in the muscles, which causes pain during and after post-workout. Post-workout stretches help to reduce lactic acid accumulation. Hydration also helps to reduce the lactic acid levels.

Post-workout stretches ensure:
- Increased flexibility
- Better posture
- Increased range of motion
- Reduced lactic acid accumulation and post-workout soreness
- Improves blood flow.

Your post-workout stretches could be 5-10 minutes after the main workout. Below are some of the post-workout stretches that can be included as per your target muscle group for the day:

Upper Body
- Cobra stretch (for upper body and lower back)
- Pec stretches (for chest)
- Shoulder stretch (for shoulder)
- Cat cow stretch (for neck, shoulder & spine)
- Child pose (for lower back muscles)
- Seated spinal twist (for upper body & hips)
- Standing biceps stretch (for biceps)
- Overhead triceps stretch (for triceps)
- Arm and wrist stretch (for arm)
- Forearm extensors stretch (for extensor muscles of forearm)
- Forearm flexors stretch (for inside muscles of forearm)

Lower Body
- Sumo squat stretch (for lower body)
- Lunging hip flexor stretch (for lower body)
- Rectus femoris stretch (for hip and knee)
- Frog stretch (for inner thighs and hips)
- Hamstring stretch (for hamstring)
- Standing quadriceps stretch (for quads)
- Standing wall calves stretch (for calves)

Chapter 7: Flexibility and Mobility

The ability of our muscles, tendons and ligaments to stretch passively is the **flexibility**. In contrast, the ability of our joints to move actively through their full range of motion is **mobility**.
We have active control over the range of motions that defines mobility, and it demands strength, control, coordination and balance, while flexibility demands how far we can stretch. It's possible for a person to have flexibility and lack mobility, as mobility also requires stability and strength.
Both are equally important since if the joints are restricted, you won't benefit much from your stretching routine. Also, if your muscles lack flexibility, it will also impact your mobility.

Apart from workouts, we also need flexibility and mobility in our daily activities, and they improve our quality of life.

Flexibility can be influenced by the following:
- Flexibility usually decreases with **age**.
- **Genes** can impact your natural flexibility.
- **Hormones** can affect the elasticity of the connective tissue.
- The female **gender** tends to be more flexible.
- Past **injuries** can impact flexibility.

Mobility can be influenced by the following factors:
- Mobility also decreases with **age**.
- Different **joint structures** and types of joints impact various movements.
- Some **medical conditions** can affect mobility.
- **More fat or more muscles** impact mobility.

A limited range of motion for an extended period can also shorten your muscles and impact your flexibility. For example, if your routine demands long hours of sitting, your hip flexors muscles could be shortened. The same could occur if you bicycle for a longer duration. Shortening of hip flexor muscles can eventually impact your shock absorbing and load bearing and capacity of the spine.

Dynamic stretching during warm-up is an effective way to work on your mobility, while static stretching post-workout would help you increase your flexibility.

High body temperature helps achieve a full range of motion and helps to improve joint flexibility; hence, warm-up is always required before performing static stretches. Passive warm-up, like a hot shower, raises only the surface temperature; therefore, active warm-up, including muscular activity, is needed to raise the core temperature.

No one likes high humidity, but as a matter of fact, humidity plays a vital role in flexibility and stretching. High humidity means you will take comparatively less time to warm up.

Breathe normally during stretching, as holding your breath increases muscular tension and blood pressure, while breathing correctly (i.e. when you exhale during elongation while stretching) could help relax the muscles.

Chapter 8: Good Body Posture and Self-Check

The musculoskeletal alignment helps in creating good body posture. Our bones and muscles are balanced if the posture is correct and our body is symmetrical. Deviation in posture usually occurs when a few muscles lack the strength to hold our body in the required position. For example, weak lower body muscles impact the posture of the trunk during standing and even sitting, and it also impacts the form while lifting weights.

You must have heard people saying you should maintain a good body posture if your work demands sitting for long hours. Still, to maintain a good posture passively, you must have musculoskeletal strength to maintain the correct posture.

If you cannot keep your trunk straight while running or if your feet or thighs are rotated outward while walking, you are prone to hip and knee joint injuries in the long run.

Proper posture also helps keep organs in place, so they work effectively and efficiently. For example, in posture deviation like swayback (where the spine curves far inwards than the normal position), the intestines are pressed against the abdominal cavity, which impacts its normal activities. Deviations like rounded shoulders and rounded upper back impact the

utilization of lungs since it doesn't allow air to be filled completely in our lungs.
So, there are external problems related to joints and internal problems that eventually occur in the long run due to bad posture.

How do you perform a self-check on your posture?

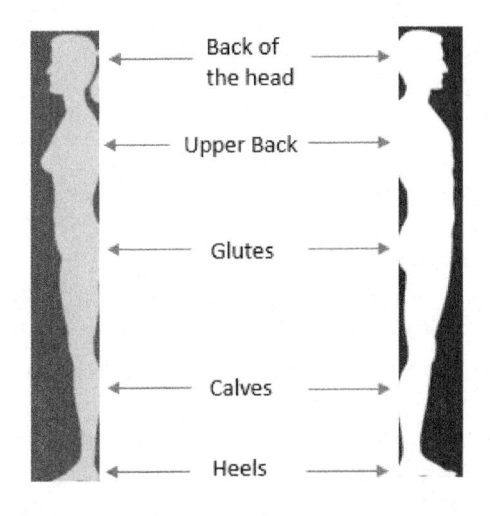

```
Back of the head
Upper Back
Glutes
Calves
Heels
```

Females – Yes, remove your scrunchies from your head before checking the posture.

Stand against the wall in such a way that your below-mentioned body parts just touch the wall, as shown in the images:
- Back of the head
- Upper back
- Glutes
- Calves
- Heels

If you need to push to make contact on any one or more parts, then there is a probability that you have some deviation.

Also, check your front view by standing straight and asking someone to click a picture from the front. Add a line right at the centre of your body, trying to divide it into two halves. If the halves are symmetrical, congratulations! Otherwise, there is a deviation if your shoulder or body is leaning to one side.

Some of the postural deviations are:
- **Swayback or Lordosis:** The inward curve of the spine is exaggerated in this condition that affects the lower back. Apart from lumber lordosis, cervical lordosis (more common in children) could also occur where the inward curve of the neck is exaggerated.
- **Scoliosis:** In this condition, there is an abnormal sideways or lateral curvature of the spine. It usually occurs before puberty; generally, the cases are mild, but in some cases, they become more severe as they grow. Scoliosis can be thoracic scoliosis (abnormal curve just below the neck), lumbar scoliosis (abnormal curve at the lower back), thoraco-lumbar scoliosis (abnormal curve from upper to lower back), combined scoliosis (abnormal curve in the opposite direction, one below the neck and other at the lower back).

- **Kyphosis:** The forward and exaggerated rounding of the upper back due to weakness in the spinal bones is termed Kyphosis.
- **Flatback:** In this deviation, the lower spine loses its normal curvature and turns flat.

Ergonomics at Workplace
- People with jobs demanding long working hours at desks should ensure that their chairs have lumbar support and armrests to reduce pressure on the discs.
- Sitting in a reclined position at approximately 120 degrees puts less pressure on discs; hence, your chairs should have the feature of alternating positions at different angles.
- Your desk set-up should allow you to open your knees if you sit longer.
- Your armrest should be placed at such an angle that your forearms should make a 90-degree angle from your upper arm. This reduces stress on the upper back and neck.

The pressure between the discs (intradiscal pressure) when sitting could be around 11 times more than when lying down.
That's the reason why short breaks are recommended after every half an hour or so with people having long sitting hours.

A strong core and lower body could help correct imbalances in muscle strength, and it keeps your body balanced by creating a strong and stable foundation. So, do not skip your leg day workout!

Chapter 9: Cardiovascular Training

Cardiovascular training is the process of exercising aerobically, where you overload the oxygen transport and utilization and eventually make your body adapt to such demands.

Cardiovascular activities increase the ability of your lungs and heart to supply oxygen-rich blood to the muscle tissues. They also increase your muscles' ability to use oxygen in order to produce energy.

Cardiovascular activities are essential to keep your heart healthy and help you live longer. The training increases your heart rate during the process and makes you breathe harder, which helps you burn body fat. Increased heart rate is an external indication of oxygen consumption.

Aerobic exercise helps relieve stress, depression, and anxiety and slows the ageing process. They also improve the quality of sleep, increase HDL and improve mental alertness. If you are getting out of breath while climbing a few stairs, it's a clear sign that you must include some cardiovascular activities in your routine.

The capacity to consume, transport and utilize oxygen is termed **aerobic fitness**.

VO2 max is the maximum rate of oxygen consumption that a person can use during a period of time.

Few myths about cardiovascular activities.

More cardio is better.
Research has shown that 4 sessions of 45 minutes each per week is sufficient, and more than that will have a limited effect on improving your aerobic capacity. If you are on muscle gain, avoid cardiovascular training for more than 90 hours per week as it could be counterproductive.

Running is the best cardiovascular activity.
The best cardio activity for you is the one that you enjoy and can continue for lifelong. It is fine to go even for a brisk walk if you have limitations in running or performing other cardiovascular activities due to age, medical condition, or obesity factors. The idea is to make your lungs and heart work harder during the process, which would also prevent the clogging of arteries with plaque.

Weight training is enough to keep yourself fit.
Resistance training is definitely a great way to keep yourself fit, but it cannot be replaced with cardiovascular activities and vice versa. Both have their own benefits, and your training schedule must include both of them to achieve maximum benefits. A person with a perfect

physique but a clogged heart cannot be called fit.

Cardio is good for the heart and lungs but not for muscles.
Cardiovascular training is not only good for heart and lungs, but it is also good for muscles as it increases the ability of our muscles to use fat as a source of energy. It also increases the size and count of mitochondria (powerhouse of cells), which helps in producing aerobic energy.

Exercise harder to improve your aerobic fitness.
It takes time for your body to adapt to the training demands, and you should not overdo it in the beginning, which could lead to injuries and demotivation. Always take it slow and steady. The process is as good as driving a vehicle steadily and safely. If you focus on speed as a beginner, you might lose control and crash your vehicle.

Cardiovascular activities make you sacrifice your joints.
While some of the cardiovascular activities could involve orthopedic trauma in case you are already struggling with your joint health, there are activities like rowing, elliptical cross trainer, and cycling, which do not put pressure on your knees.

There are ample cardiovascular activities and equipment that can be used for cardiovascular training as per the intensity level.

A beginner can start by adding walk if your existing schedule is completely sedentary. However, remember that walking has the least effect on aerobic fitness level as it does not raise your heart zone to the training zone, so your goal should be to improve your cardiovascular stamina gradually. This does not seem possible once on the first day, but don't get disheartened. Your stamina improves with time if you are consistent.
Add a few bursts of brisk walk while walking. If you have access to a gym, you can add cycling, elliptical cross trainer, rowing, or treadmill walk/jog. Zumba and other dance training can also be included if you like it.

Gradually, with time, you can increase the intensity of your training to improve your cardiovascular stamina, and you can also go for jumping activities once your weight management is in control and you do not have any limitations or medical conditions. You can also go for any sport or HIIT.

HIIT (High Intensity Interval Training)
Recent studies have shown that HIIT works better than static and conventional cardiovascular activities like running on a treadmill or cycling.
HIIT or High-Intensity Interval Training is an intense exercise of short bursts alternated recovery periods of low-intensity, like 20 seconds of intense exercise followed by 10 seconds of rest and so on.

20-30 minutes HIIT session is draining enough, and it increases your metabolic rate for hours, accounting for more EPOC as compared to other light to moderate intensity workouts. HIIT may improve VO2 max, which means the heart and lungs are able to deliver more oxygen to muscles. HIIT can also increase testosterone, as per some studies.

HIIT is more effective, but it can also be a little taxing to beginners and people having some back or neck pain problems since the intensity of the program pushes you to an extent where you could lose your form after a few cycles if your stamina doesn't allow you to stay in the game till the end.

The buzz around - 'High-intensity workouts are harmful'.
This cannot be concluded in general. If you are already a heart patient or have hypertension, you must avoid high-intensity workouts. Doing that can put more pressure on your heart, which is already weak.
If you are starting your training in your teenage or in your early 20s, it is a great time to make your heart stronger. In general, if you have grown older without any cardiovascular activity, you need to level up your intensity of the workout gradually rather than putting too much pressure on your heart for a longer duration of time instantly as a beginner. A few heart attacks you hear about while performing high-intensity activities or during marathons are examples of either improper training or

putting too much pressure on your heart for a longer duration of time for which the heart was not appropriately trained.

A heart rate beyond 90% of the maximum heart rate for a longer duration, like an hour or more, is an example of putting unnecessary pressure on the heart than needed in normal scenarios. So, maintain a heart rate between 55%-85% of the maximum heart rate (Maximum heart rate = 220 – Your age).

Do not compare normal scenarios with the training schedule of professional athletes. They start their training at a very early age, and they train their heart, body, and mind to that level gradually.

Chapter 10: Resistance Training

Resistance training
Resistance training is a form of training that increases strength and endurance. The training causes our muscles to contract against resistance. Some of the major kinds of resistance include:
- **Body weight** workouts like push-ups, pull-ups, and squats are a kind of resistance training where your own weight acts as resistance while performing these exercises. As a beginner, you can always start with body-weight workouts at home.
- **Variable resistance** includes resistance bands and machines where resistance varies during the movement. There are exercises that don't lend themselves to training with free weights. Here, such variable resistance training machines give an edge. However, the major disadvantage is that the movement in such machines is unnatural, so the surrounding muscles are not under tension, and hence, they don't get strengthened, unlike the case in free-weight training.
- **Constant resistance** includes training with barbells and dumbbells where the resistance is constant. This is natural and more effective in longer duration, but for a beginner, you could struggle a bit in the beginning with the form.

- **Accommodating resistance** includes machines like treadmills or stationary cycles where you can control the speed and exert maximum resistance during the entire range of motion. Unlike variable resistance, the resistance is constant here during a range of motion, but you can vary resistance by controlling speed, which can't be done in constant resistance equipment.
- **Static resistance** workouts include isometric exercises where the muscle length is constant during a contraction. For example, if you hold a squat position, a plank position, or you hold a barbell during a curl for a few seconds, it is an isometric movement. But we need to become stronger during the entire range of motion, which is restricted by static resistance.

What kind of resistance training should you go for?

All kinds of resistance training have some pros and cons, and it's best to use their pros to our advantage by including most or all of them in our training plan.

Your cardiovascular training could include treadmill, elliptical or stationary cycles, which have accommodating resistance. If you are a beginner, you should start with body-weight workouts and machine workouts, as machines provide safety support and a form check to some extent. Gradually, after two or three weeks, when your form and strength improve, you can start including more free-weight workouts than machines, but it is still a good idea to have both in your workout plan.

Muscle failure is a stage where you cannot perform one more complete repetition without support. We must target muscle failure gradually since this puts more tension on our muscle fibers, recruits a maximum number of motor units and hence maximizes muscle growth.

Are free weights better than Smith machines for workouts?
It depends! The Smith machine is great for workouts when you want to focus on the primary muscles since the bar in the machine follows the guided path, and hence, there is less use of assistance muscles. Also, you can perform reps till muscle failure since it has a great safety mechanism.
Free weights are good for maximizing the overall muscle strength, including primary and assistance muscles, but there are certain exercises in which performing reps till muscle failure could be risky, and you might need a spotter, like a bench press.
It is a good practice to include a Smith machine as well as free weight workouts and alternate times for a muscle group.

How much weight should you lift?
This again depends on your goal, but considering you are a beginner and have no idea how much you should lift. You will have to

do some hit and trial initially. Start with the minimum weight with which you feel you can do 12-15 repetitions (rep) and perform around 3 sets. Remember that initially, your form is more important than how much you are lifting. If your form is going wrong after a few reps, you are lifting more than you should.

Also, after the first day, it is natural to feel muscle soreness, which is also called as DOMS (Delayed Onset Muscle Soreness), and it could persist for 36-72 hours. If your pain persists for more than 72 hours, it means you overdid it. To get relief from the soreness, you can apply an ice pack on the sore area post-workout.

Do not skip your workout because you have soreness. You might feel that you won't be able to perform any exercise the next day, but after warm-up and dynamic stretches, you might feel a little better.

After a week, if you are able to perform 15-20 or more repetitions with the correct form and your soreness is under control, you can increase your weight slightly to the extent that you can perform 12-15 reps with the right form.

After another 2-3 weeks, when you feel that you are able to perform the required reps easily, keeping the form intact, then you can go for weights where your muscle failure would arrive in 12-15 reps, but as a beginner, if you are reaching the level of muscle failure, you must have a spotter in workouts where safety mechanism is not present, or you can perform those workout over machines for safety reasons. Hitting failure in every set is not required in the beginning. You can start with one set per exercise per muscle group, where you can take the reps till failure, keeping safety measures in mind.

As per our goal, our reps and sets may vary. The below table suggests a generic rep range and set range as per goal, which is mostly followed in the fitness industry.

Goal	Repetitions	Sets
Power	1-2	3-5
Strength	3-6	2-6
Hypertrophy	6-12	3-6
Endurance	12+	2-3

Hypertrophy is increase in muscle size. You can still increase muscle size if your rep range is of power, strength or endurance. It is just that the ratio of hypertrophy will differ as per the rep range and it will be maximum in the range of 6-12 reps.

The repetition range mentioned in the above table means that your muscle failure should come in that range, which indirectly means that you need to choose such weights while doing the sets. So, if you are training for hypertrophy, you must lift weights in such a way that you should be able to perform at least 3 sets of minimum 6 reps each. If you are unable to complete those 6 reps or unable to complete those 3 sets, you are lifting heavier than you should. Similarly, if you are able to lift more than 12 reps, you are lifting lighter than you should lift for your goal.

1 RM – 1 Rep Max
One rep max is the maximum weight you can lift for only one repetition with the correct form. As a beginner, you don't need to do 1RM in your workout, but knowing one rep max allows you to select the right weight for your exercise to maximize your training and increase your strength gradually.
The powerlifters in the Olympics perform 1RM that you see on television.

Several calculations and workout plans are designed based on your one rep max, and to know your one rep max, you should pick a weight with which you reach failure in 6-12 reps.
For example, if you choose:
60 kg weight and perform 8 reps on a bench press, then as per the below chart, 8 reps means you have hit 80% of one rep max, and hence, according to the basic math, the calculation for your one rep max is here:
80% of X = 60 (where X = 1RM)
X = 75 kg = 1RM.

Rep Count	Maximum Percentage
12	70
11	72.5
10	75
9	77.5

8	80
7	82.5
6	85
5	87.5
4	90
3	92.5
2	95
1	100

Chapter 11: Muscle Contractions & ATP-ADP Cycle

There are three main types of muscle contractions:
- **Concentric contraction:** Lifting a weight that contracts the primary muscles is called concentric contraction or positive movement. This is also known as the overcoming phase. E.g., Lifting up a dumbbell in a dumbbell curl.
- **Eccentric contraction:** Lowering a weight where primary muscle length increases is called eccentric contraction or negative movement. This is also known as the yielding phase. E.g., Lowering down the dumbbell in dumbbell curl.
- **Isometric contraction:** Holding a weight where muscle length is constant is called isometric contraction. E.g., Holding a dumbbell up in a static position during a dumbbell curl after concentric movement.

While performing any workout, your eccentric movement should not go with the flow of gravity. You must resist the flow to feel the tension.

If you are on hypertrophy, eccentric training should be in your recipe. We can lift 1.6X more weights on an eccentric movement than concentric movement. Even if you get muscle failure on concentric movement, you must try to get support on concentric movement and perform your reps to get an eccentric failure. This will help you increase muscle mass.

Terms you might hear from fitness experts – Agonist and Antagonist
The agonist is the muscle that is contracting, and the antagonist is the muscle that is relaxing. Example: During biceps curl, biceps are agonists, and triceps are antagonists.

ATP & ADP Cycle

ATP: Adenosine Triphosphate
ADP: Adenosine Diphosphate

During exercise, ATP is broken down by our cells to ADP (Adenosine Diphosphate), a phosphate molecule and energy is released.

ATP -> ADP + P (Energy released for cells)

ADP is then further converted to ATP by adding inorganic phosphate molecules with the help of the enzyme ATP synthase.

ADP + P -> ATP (Energy absorbed from food)

High-intensity or explosive workouts need more ATP each second than our body can produce.

Have you ever wondered why world-class sprinters start panting in 10-15 seconds while marathoners do not? Sprinting is an explosive workout, while long-distance running is an endurance sport where we do not go all out for the entire duration. All such explosive sport like sprinting and powerlifting needs ATP, and in maximal efforts, ATP is totally gone within 1.26 seconds!

In powerlifting or any explosive activity, 3 minutes of rest is normal since the ATP that has been depleted needs approximately this much time to replenish the new ones.

In weight training, concentric muscle contractions need more ATP than eccentric contraction.

We will discuss more about this cycle under 'Creatine' section of supplements.

Chapter 12: Training Techniques and Principles

There are several training methods and principles. Almost all of them have worked on subjects and proven beneficial under certain conditions. You might see different techniques being followed by different people in the gym. No technique or principle is right or wrong. You just need to find out which works best for you and could fit into your schedule. You always have the choice to switch to other training methods and principles if you feel your progress is stagnant, and also the change will add flavour to your existing schedule.

Let's discuss some of the most common methods that can be included in your workout schedule for greater gains.

Technique	Description	To be used by
Beyond Failure	Once you reach concentric failure, take support on concentric movement from a partner if available and perform 2-3 more reps. In these reps, take	Intermediate/ Advanced

	4-6 seconds to perform eccentric movement so that you reach eccentric failure too. *(Partner needed for to implement this properly)*	
Tempo Training	Complete the concentric movement in 1 second and take around 4 seconds for the eccentric movement.	Beginner/ Intermediate/ Advanced
Negative Overload	Start your set with the maximum weight, perform one eccentric movement and let your partner provide full support to perform the	Advanced

	concentric movement you reach eccentric failure. Eg: Start your bench press with maximum weight (1RM) and lower the weight (eccentric movement), let your partner lift the weight back to the top position from where you start lower the weight again. *(Partner needed to implement this properly)*	
2 Up – 1 Down	Lift the weight (concentric) using both the hands and lower down (eccentric) using one hand. If you are able to perform concentric	Intermediate/ Advanced

	movement of the set with one hand as well, then the weight is not enough.	
Rest Pause	Take 85%-95% of your one rep-max and then take 15-30 seconds' rest. Repeat it until failure with the same weight. Another variation could be to use a weight with which you can perform 6-10 reps to reach failure. Rest for 15 seconds and repeat the process until failure. This time you might be able to perform 3-4 reps and next time 2-3 reps after 15	Advanced

	seconds' rest. Repeat this till failure.	
German Volume Training	Since volume = reps * sets * weight and to achieve hypertrophy, we need higher volume for more gains. As per German volume training theory, we need to attack the same muscles with 10 sets. Eg: Perform 10 sets of bench press with 10 reps each with the moderate weight with which you will be able to complete all the sets and reps. In case, you are unable to complete the last	Beginner/ Intermediate/ Advanced

	reps of a set, reduce the weight by ~5%. You must target 2-3 muscles groups in parallel while using this technique like Shoulder Press (10 sets *10 reps), Chin-ups (10 sets *10 reps) and Crunches (10 sets *10 reps).	
Pre-exhaustion Technique	This is a conventional technique which says that if we perform single-joint muscle to failure followed by compound movement, it will recruit more muscle fiber because muscle failure will occur	Advanced

	before neurological failure, and this will result in more muscle gains. However, a study in 2003 in the *'Journal of Strength and Conditioning Research' conducted on 17 men* proved that the failure of single joint muscles leads to reduced strength in performing compound movement later which is the core of our training.	
Post-exhaustion Technique	This is the most common training style where compound movements are performed first followed by	Beginner/ Intermediate/ Advanced

	isolation muscle movements. This allows more strength during the core compound movements followed by isolation workouts for better muscular gains.	
Cheating	Complete the concentric movement with a swing and perform the controlled eccentric movement. This means you are cheating on concentric movements to reach eccentric failure. So, the technique is equivalent to negative overload without	Advanced

	a partner. Another variation could be to use this technique once you reach the concentric failure. Eg: After reaching concentric failure in barbell curl, swing the bar upwards and from the top position, lower the weight (eccentric) slowly to reach eccentric failure. Beginners should avoid it as it could mess up their form if you are already struggling with form initially.	
Muscle Confusion	On continuously applying the same tension, your muscles get	Intermediate/ Advanced

	adapt to it and hinders the growth. This technique demands change in sets, reps, exercises, movement speed, weights and attacking the muscles from different angles.	
Superset Training	Training opposing muscle groups alternately, but do not compromise with the training intensity and you can rest for both the muscle groups as well. More work in less time. Eg: Chest and Back, Shoulders and Legs (like performing 1 set of bench press	Intermediate/ Advanced

	and then 1 set of seated machine row, and repeat)	
Compound Sets	Performing two exercises alternately for one muscle group with minimal rest between sets. Eg: Preacher curl followed by dumbbell hammer curl	Intermediate/ Advanced
Staggered Sets	Training small and slow developing muscles in between larger muscle groups. Eg: Wrist curl in between leg extension.	Beginner / Intermediate/ Advanced
Pyramid Training	This is a traditional technique where we increase the load in every set (light to heavy) until we reach	Beginner / Intermediate/ Advanced

	the one rep max	
Reverse Pyramid Training	Here we start our set with maximum load (after warm-up) and perform set till failure, decrease the load (by ~20%) after each set, take some rest and repeat.	Intermediate/ Advanced
Drop Sets	This is like reverse pyramid technique, but there should be no to minimum rest between sets.	Intermediate/ Advanced
Quality Training	Decreasing the rest periods between sets and increasing or maintaining the reps every set.	Beginner / Intermediate/ Advanced
Continuous Tension	Maintaining slow and continuous movement	Intermediate/ Advanced

	without letting the muscles to relax in a set (like not taking rest at the top of the certain movements). Eg: In a bench press, slowly lift the bar up, and just when are about to reach the top, start taking the bar down gradually in order to maintain continuous tension.	
Partial Reps	As per this technique, since leverage changes throughout the exercise, partial movement can be performed in a few reps with increased load to attain maximum overload stress	Advanced

	on a muscle which is restricted in full range of motion. (*This technique should only be applied for the last few reps and not as a whole, unless you are training professionally with a goal as performing half range of motion could impact your flexibility.*)	
5*5 Technique	It involves 5 sets * 5 reps with a constant weight to gain strength in compound movements. You should use 75-80% of your one rep-max (means you should be able to do 7-8 reps of that load to reach failure).	Beginner / Intermediate/ Advanced

In the above table, levels cannot be the same for everyone but let's try to understand how we can categorize someone when it comes to choosing techniques.

- ➢ Beginner level: You have just started resistance training and still struggling with forms for most of the workout.
- ➢ Intermediate level: It's been more than six months since you have started working out regularly and you are not at all struggling with form and basic techniques for all the workouts.
- ➢ Advanced level: You have been regularly training for over a year or more and you are able to perform all the workouts with the perfect form and different techniques. You have shown decent progress in terms of strength and body composition and do not have any medical condition or injury.

Chapter 13: Strength Workouts for Major Muscle Groups

Now, the exercises that we are going to discuss below are the common ones for which you must find videos on the internet, and you can go through them to check the form. I know that's some effort if you really have no clue about these workouts. Please do that effort for yourself! It's just a one-time effort and you will definitely find reference for them easily.

Also, for the first month, if you can afford, you can hire a personal trainer to get your form corrected and push you through the workouts.

MUSCLE Map

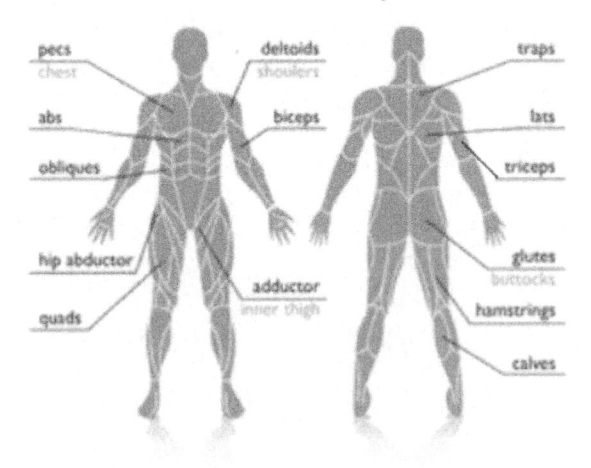

pecs — chest
deltoids — shoulders
abs
biceps
obliques
traps
lats
triceps
hip abductor
adductor — inner thigh
quads
glutes — buttocks
hamstrings
calves

Front View   Back View

Muscle Group	Exercise
Chest	Wide Hand Push Ups
	Flat Bench Press - Barbell/Dumbbell
	Butterfly Press
	Inclined Bench Press – Barbell/Dumbbell
	Inclined Bench Dumbbell Flyes
	Chest Bar Dips
	Cable Crossovers
	Decline Bench Press – Barbell/Dumbbell
Lats	Pull Ups/ Lat Pull Down
	Chin Ups
	Seated Machine Row
	Barbell Bent Over Row
	Single Arm Dumbbell Row
Trapezius	Reverse Fly
	Shrugs – Barbell/Dumbbell/Cable Bar
Deltoids	Shoulder Press
	Dumbbell Press
	Barbell Upright Row
	Dumbbell Posterior Deltoid Raise
	Lateral Raise
	Single Arm Cable Posterior

	Deltoid Raise
Triceps	Triceps Dips
	Dumbbell Triceps Extension
	Triceps Kickbacks
	Triceps Cable Extension
	Triceps Pushdown
	Reverse Pushdowns
Biceps	Barbell/Dumbbell Curl
	Cable Biceps Curl
	Hammer Curl
	Concentration Curl
Abdomen	Crunches
	Butterfly Crunches
	Bicycle Crunches
	Lying Leg Raises
	Reverse Crunches
Rotator Cuff Muscles	Lying Dumbbell Horizontal External Rotation
	Seated Dumbbell Horizontal External Rotation
	External Rotation at 90 Degree Abduction
Legs	Squats
	Deadlift
	Barbell/Dumbbell Squats
	Front Squats
	Leg Press
	Leg Extension

	Lunges
	Leg Curl
Calf	Seated Calf Raise
	Standing Weighted Calf Raise
Glutes	Hip Thrusts
	Deadlift & Sumo-Deadlift
	Bulgarian Split Squats
	Single Leg Deadlift

There are many muscles in a single muscle group. We are discussing workouts for muscle group as a whole to avoid the discussions around anatomy and scientific names which would be too much information for a beginner.

Exercises like push-ups, pull-ups, squats, deadlifts, bench presses, overhead/shoulder presses, and dips are some of the compound movements that target more than one muscle group. You should include more compound movement workouts than isolation movement workouts in your schedule as compound movements:
- Burn more calories
- Improve overall strength
- Improve intramuscular coordination
- Improve flexibility and mobility
- Rapid muscle growth

Chapter 14: How to Prepare Your Workout Plan?: Gym & Home Workout

To prepare your workout plan, you need to take care of the following factors in order:
- Goal
- Frequency
- Equipment
- Split
- Technique
- Exercises
- Volume

Goal
You should be clear about what you want to achieve.
- Muscle Gain: You are on a calorie surplus diet and can focus on hypertrophy, strength, power or endurance. Try to hit muscle failure while performing reps of exercises. Focus more on eccentric movements.
- Fat Loss: This is a calorie deficit phase, and hence, your nutrition and workout should be balanced in order to avoid being too low on energy.
- Maintenance: This is a decent phase to focus on achieving a little more muscle mass and losing a little more fat mass if needed. You can focus on improving

strength, power or endurance in this phase as well.

Frequency
How many days of the week can you workout?
- Beginners: They can target 4-5 days a week for 45-60 minutes sessions per day.
- Intermediate: They can target 5-6 days a week for a 60-minute session per day.
- Advanced: They can target 6 days a week for 75-90 minute sessions per day.
- Elite or Professional: They can target even 10+ sessions a week for 60-90 minutes session per day or as per your goal.

The above information is to give you an idea about how most people plan their workouts, but frequency is something that cannot be fixed as per the above data. We need to figure out how many days and how much time per day we can devote to our training in the beginning. Also, our stamina in the beginning might not allow us to complete 60 minutes, which is absolutely fine. We need to plan our workouts accordingly, even if we are in the game for 30 minutes initially. If we are unable to complete the workouts daily, even after pushing, that means our plan needs to be updated. With time, the stamina will improve, and you will be able to perform 60 minutes of workout.

Equipment
Do you have access to a gym, or will you start with home workouts?

If you are starting with a home workout, do you have any equipment? Dumbbells, barbells or kettlebells?
If not, then we need to choose the home workouts accordingly. Some home workouts are shared under the 'Exercises' section of this chapter.

Split
According to the number of days, a split should be planned.

<u>4 days in a week</u>

Days	Split
Monday	Upper Body
Tuesday	Lower Body
Wednesday	Rest
Thursday	Upper Body
Friday	Lower Body
Saturday	Rest
Sunday	Rest

Alternatively, you can also start with lower body first. It doesn't make any difference.

Days	Split
Monday	Push (Chest, Shoulders, Triceps)
Tuesday	Pull (Back & Biceps)
Wednesday	Rest

Thursday	Legs & Core
Friday	Cardio/ Calisthenics/ Yoga/ Full Body/ Martial Arts/ Sports, etc.
Saturday	Rest
Sunday	Rest

Pushing resistance is a positive movement in the chest, shoulders and triceps; we push the barbell upwards in the chest and shoulder press and push the bar or rope downwards in a triceps pushdown workout.

Similarly, pulling a resistance is a positive movement in the back and biceps, like in lat pull-down or pulling the resistance upwards in a barbell or dumbbell curl.

Days	Split
Monday	Full Body
Tuesday	Rest
Wednesday	Cardio/ Calisthenics/ Yoga/ Martial Arts/ Sports, etc.
Thursday	Rest
Friday	Lower Body
Saturday	Rest
Sunday	Cardio/ Calisthenics/ Yoga/ Martial Arts/ Sports, etc.

Days	Split
Monday	Full Body

Tuesday	Rest
Wednesday	Full Body
Thursday	Rest
Friday	Full Body
Saturday	Rest
Sunday	Cardio

<u>5 days in a week</u>

Days	Split
Monday	Upper Body
Tuesday	Lower Body
Wednesday	Rest
Thursday	Upper Body
Friday	Lower Body
Saturday	Rest
Sunday	Cardio

Rest days can be managed as per your convenience.

Days	Split
Monday	Push (Chest, Shoulders, Triceps)
Tuesday	Pull (Back & Biceps)
Wednesday	Legs
Thursday	Rest
Friday	Cardio/ Calisthenics/ Yoga/ Martial Arts / Sports, etc.
Saturday	Cardio/ Calisthenics/ Yoga/

	Martial Arts / Sports, etc.
Sunday	Rest

Alternatively, if you are more into yoga, sports, calisthenics, martial arts, etc., you can do that 3 days a week and do either push and pull for 2 days or upper body for two days with a rest day in between.

Days	Split
Monday	Push (Chest, Shoulders, Triceps)
Tuesday	Pull (Back & Biceps)
Wednesday	Legs
Thursday	Rest
Friday	Upper Body
Saturday	Lower Body
Sunday	Rest

6 days in a week

Days	Split
Monday	Upper Body
Tuesday	Lower Body
Wednesday	Upper Body
Thursday	Lower Body
Friday	Upper Body
Saturday	Lower Body
Sunday	Rest

Days	Split
Monday	Push (Chest, Shoulders, Triceps)
Tuesday	Pull (Back & Biceps)
Wednesday	Legs
Thursday	Push (Chest, Shoulders, Triceps)
Friday	Pull (Back & Biceps)
Saturday	Legs
Sunday	Rest

Days	Split
Monday	Chest & Triceps
Tuesday	Back & Biceps
Wednesday	Legs & Shoulders
Thursday	Chest & Triceps
Friday	Back & Biceps
Saturday	Legs & Shoulders
Sunday	Rest

Days	Split
Monday	Chest & Back
Tuesday	Shoulders, Biceps & Triceps
Wednesday	Legs & Core
Thursday	Chest & Back
Friday	Shoulders, Biceps & Triceps
Saturday	Legs & Core
Sunday	Rest

Above is the opposing muscles workout plan where chest and back, biceps and triceps, quadriceps and hamstrings are the opposing muscles and the other muscle group rests while performing exercise for one muscle group. For example, if you are doing bench press, it will impact your chest muscles but not your back muscles, and hence, it will lead to quicker recovery between workouts and also reduce muscle fatigue during the training session.

Days	Split
Monday	Push (Chest, Shoulders, Triceps)
Tuesday	Cardio/ Calisthenics/ Yoga/ Martial Arts / Sports, etc.
Wednesday	Pull (Back & Biceps)
Thursday	Cardio/ Calisthenics/ Yoga/ Martial Arts / Sports, etc.
Friday	Legs
Saturday	Cardio/ Calisthenics/ Yoga/ Martial Arts / Sports, etc.
Sunday	Rest

Days	Split
Monday	Cardio/ Calisthenics/ Yoga/ Martial Arts/ Sports, etc.
Tuesday	Cardio/ Calisthenics/ Yoga/ Martial Arts / Sports, etc.

Wednesday	Upper Body
Thursday	Cardio/ Calisthenics/ Yoga/ Martial Arts / Sports, etc.
Friday	Cardio/ Calisthenics/ Yoga/ Martial Arts / Sports, etc.
Saturday	Lower Body
Sunday	Rest

So, the split can be created as per the number of days you are going to workout and your interest in the kind of physical activities you want to choose. If your sports or activity includes resistance training session(s) for different muscle groups, that's great! But remember, the physical activity should not just be cardio for the entire week, else you will not gain strength and muscle mass and ultimately lose metabolism. Also, now we know that only cardio will not help us in getting the cuts and perfect shape that you are looking for.

Things to Remember
- Start your workout with a bigger muscle group if you are training multiple muscle groups in a day.
- Chest and back are the biggest muscle groups in the upper body, followed by shoulders and then biceps and triceps. If it is your push day, start with chest workouts. Ample bigger muscle workouts are compound movements (like

bench presses, squats, deadlifts, and shoulder presses).

- When you are training for a bigger muscle group like the chest, your smaller muscles like shoulders, triceps and biceps are also being worked out to some extent due to compound movements. Similarly, a workout for the back warms up and trains your biceps muscle group and movements like deadlift train your posterior chain, including glutes, quadriceps, hamstrings and other leg muscles.
- Target each muscle group twice a week for hypertrophy.
- Plan your split in such a way that every muscle group gets 48 hours of rest to recover before you train that muscle group again.
- Do not choose similar movements on machines and free weights as different exercises on the same day. For example, the Bench press and dumbbell press are similar movements, and the shoulder press using a barbell and dumbbell is another example of similar movement. Alternatively, perform them in a week if you are planning to hit one muscle group twice a week.
- If you feel there are too many exercises to do on one day when we hit more than one muscle group, you are right, but you can still perform the same number of sets you would have done with a single muscle group with a limited number of

exercises. For example, Perform bench press, inclined bench press and butterfly press for chest one day, and push-ups, decline bench press and cable crossovers on the other day of the week. This way, you will hit the mid and upper chest on one day while the mid and lower chest on the other day.

➢ You don't need a supporter or a belt if you are increasing your level gradually, as that will make your core stronger with time. If you are into powerlifting or lifting beyond your own weight, you can use a belt that will help you to keep your core intact and maintain form to some extent, through which you can focus on lifting more. Remember that rule number 1 is always to focus on form before you increase the weight.

➢ Do not wear gym belts throughout the session. By doing so, you are not helping your back and core to get stronger, which could affect your daily life activities in case you need to lift heavy luggage. Use a belt only for heavy weights when you feel it is getting difficult to keep your core intact.

➢ No matter how pro you become, always use safety racks while performing movements like squats and similarly, get a spotter if you are going beyond limits in movements like bench presses. You cannot afford to hit the failure in such movements without safety measures.

Technique
Choose any technique from the training techniques and principles section as per your level. You can start with the pyramid training as a beginner, which is the most common one and choosing a lesser weight in the initial sets also warms up that muscle group.

Exercises

Warm up as per your target muscle group for the day.
Always start with a warm-up, as we discussed in the earlier chapters, which could include jogging over a treadmill for 4-5 minutes, followed by some dynamic stretches and mobility workouts.

Your dynamic stretches should focus more on the muscle groups that you are training for the day. Here are some basic dynamic stretches as per muscle groups (videos of which can be found on the internet):

- Chest & Shoulders: Arm circles, arm crossovers, dynamic, open arm chest stretch, shoulder rolls.
- Back: Torso twist, toe touch, overhead reach, standing bicycle.
- Lower Body: Leg swings, sideways leg swings, standing hip circles, body-weight squats, walking lunges.
- Biceps & Triceps: In case you are not targeting these muscle groups with chest, back or shoulders, you can pick an empty barbell and perform 2 sets of

barbell curls with 25-30 reps each for biceps and the same with overhead triceps extension for triceps.

Main workout

How many exercises per muscle group should you perform?

As a beginner, you can target 4-6 different exercises with 3 sets per exercise, which means a total of 12-18 sets. Gradually, the number of exercises can be increased after 2-3 weeks, or so once you gain some strength and stamina. Below are a few home workout exercises for each muscle group in case you do not have access to any equipment. You can choose the workouts from the below table to create your own plan.

Body weight workouts – Home workout (Start with 3 sets: 12-15 reps/set)

Muscle Group	Exercise
Chest	Wide hand Push-ups or Knee assisted push-ups *(for mid-chest)*
	Decline push-ups or Knee assisted push-ups *(for upper chest)*
	Incline push-ups *(for lower chest)*
	Archer Push ups *(for*

	intermediate to advanced level)
Shoulders	Push-ups (with hands shoulder width apart), with knee assistance if required
	Plank shoulder tap
	Plank up-and-downs
Triceps	Triceps Dips
	Diamond or close hand push-ups (with knee assistance if required)
Back	Pulls Ups/Inverted row (if possible)
	Superman Y
	Reverse snow angel
	Plank row
Biceps	Chin-ups/Inverted row (if possible)
	Towel curl
	Towel hammer curl
Legs	Squats
	Sumo squats
	Lunges variation (Forward lunges, Backward lunges, side lunges, static lunges)
	Calf Raise
Abs & Core	Crunches (Butterfly crunches, C crunches, jack-knife, V crunches)
	Leg raises

	Reverse crunches
	Bicycle crunches
	Mountain Climbers

For cardiovascular activities, apart from cycling, treadmill, elliptical cross trainers and other gym equipment, below are some of the exercises that can be included as a part of your functional or cross-fit training. You can also use some of these workouts and create your HIIT plan (20:10, 30:15 or whatever works for you).

You might not know some of the below exercises by name, but you will easily find their videos on the internet. Only perform those workouts in the beginning where you feel your form is going right without much exertion on your back or neck.

Spot Jump	Jumping Jacks
Spot Jog	Fast Feet
High Knee	Split Jacks
Overhead Arm Press	Plank
Butt Kickers	Plank Jack
High Knee with Punches	Chest Expander
Plank Shoulder Tap	Criss Cross Jacks
Panther Shoulder Tap	Alternate Arm Raise in Plank Position
Mountain Climbers Cross Body	Crab Crawl

Jumping Oblique Twist	Half Crunches
Flutter Kicks	Cross Flutter Kicks
Lying Leg Rotation	Triceps Dips
Forward Jump	Arm Circles
Wall Sit	Alternate Heel Touch
Plank Leg Raise	Side to Side Jump
Reverse Plank Hold	Glute Bridge
Seal Jacks	Glute Bridge March
Left Side Plank	Right Side Plank
Belly Penguins	Bear Walk
Beginner Russian Twist	Sprawl
Dynamic Lunges	Burpees
Basketball Squats	Duck Walk
Bird Dog	Frog Jump
Jackknife	Inchworm

Once you get used to your body weight, workouts might not challenge you after a few weeks or months. You need to increase the intensity by taking shorter breaks, or you can use weights. If you don't want to buy weights, use objects like water bottles (1 liter), bags, or any grocery packet of 5 or 10Kgs, etc. and use them in workouts like weighted squats, weighted lunges, biceps curls, weighted shoulder press, weighted triceps extension, weighted chest press.

You will find ways if you really want to achieve something.

Below are some of the workouts that can be included, along with body-weight workouts if you have dumbbells at home.

Dumbbell workouts – Home workout
(Start with 3 sets: 12-15 reps/set)

Muscle Group	Exercise
Chest	Dumbbell Chest Press (on floor)
	Lying Dumbbell Flyes
	Incline Dumbbell Press (if possible)
Shoulders	Shoulder Dumbbell Press
	Arnold Press
	Shoulder Front Raise
	Lateral Raise
Triceps	Triceps Extension
	Lying Dumbbell Triceps Extension
	Triceps Kickback
Back	Dumbbell Row/ Dumbbell Pullover
	Dumbbell Shrugs
	Dumbbell Y Raises
	Gorilla Row
Biceps	Dumbbell Curls
	Concentration Curls
	Hammer Curls
	Inverted Dumbbell Curls

Legs	Dumbbell Raise Romanian Deadlift
	Sumo Dumbbell Deadlift
	Weighted Lunges variation (Forward lunges, Backward lunges, side lunges, static lunges)
	Weighted Calf Raise

You can also go for **resistance bands**, which are quite reasonable and are also used in physical therapies during injuries. They offer variable resistance, and multiple resistance workouts can be performed from them as they provide safety door armor. Below are some of the workouts that can be performed with resistance bands:

Resistance band(s) workouts – Home workout (Start with 3 sets: 12-15 reps/set)

Muscle Group	Exercise
Chest	Chest Flyes (anchor attached at mid-level for mid-chest)
	Inclined Chest Flyes (anchor at the bottom)
	Decline Chest Flyes (anchor at the top)
Shoulders	Shoulder Press
	Shoulder Front Raise

	Lateral Raise
	Face Pull
	Internal Rotation (for rotator cuff muscles)
	External Rotation (for rotator cuff muscles)
Triceps	Triceps Extension
	Triceps Pushdown
	Triceps Kickback
	Reverse Triceps Pushdown
Back	Pull Apart
	Bend Over Row
	Superman Band Rows
Biceps	Biceps Curls
	Concentration Curls
	Hammer Curls
	Inverted Curls
Legs	Resistance Deadlift
	Weighted Squats
	Weighted Lunges variation (Forward lunges, Backward lunges, side lunges, static lunges)
	Hip Abduction (with ankle support)
	Hip Adduction (with ankle support)
	Lying Hamstring Curl (with ankle support)

If you have access to the gym, we already have the table and some workouts from which you can select 2-3 exercises per muscle group and perform 12-15 reps per set in the first few weeks.

Volume

Volume = Sets * Reps * Weight
We know the number of sets and reps. The weight cannot be constant for everyone. As we already discussed, we need to choose such weights at the beginning with which we can complete our workout. Gradually, if you feel the weights do not challenge you anymore, increase the weights in each set like in the pyramid technique. If your goal is hypertrophy, you should definitely target to increase the volume every two weeks or so.

Rest between sets and exercises

This cannot be constant and could vary from 30 seconds to 3 minutes. If you are doing high-intensity workouts like HIIT (High-Intensity Interval Training), the rest could be as low as 10-15 seconds. In resistance training, rest could be measured as when one can catch their breath in such a way that they are not cooled down to get out of their training zone and can perform the next set with the expected number of reps in a challenging way.

Do you know?
There are two types of skeletal muscle fibers in our body. Slow twitch muscle fibers and fast twitch muscle fibers. Slow twitch muscle fibers support long-distance endurance activities like a marathon, while fast twitch support explosive activities where power generation is the key, like powerlifting, sprinting, and boxing.

Chapter 15: Periodization

Periodization is mainly needed for intermediate to advanced athletes, but we should understand the concept of overreaching and overtraining to avoid performance drops and injuries.
In periodization, training is broken down into the following time periods:
- Macrocycles: Long training periods from six months to one year
- Mesocycles: Moderate training periods like a month to a few months
- Microcycles: Shortest training period lasting for a week

"The need for different phases of training is influenced by physiology because neuromuscular and cardiorespiratory development and perfection...are achieved progressively over a long period of time. One also has to consider the client's physiological and psychological potential and that athletic shape cannot be maintained throughout the year at a high level."
~ Tudor O. Bompa (Theory and Methodology of Training 1983)

Through periodization, you will also prevent injuries and overtraining, and your regimen will also not be boring.

Without periodization, you might reach the stage of overreaching and overtraining if your training is intense for a longer duration of period.

Overreaching: It is a short-term stage where your performance is decreased, and the restoration of performance could take some days to weeks.

Overtraining: It is a long-term stage where your performance is decreased, and the restoration of performance could take some weeks to months.

Research shows that training for more than 3-4 hours per day for 5-6 days a week without proper progression could also reach to such stages, while training limited to 60-90 minutes can provide greater benefits. A lot of endurance athletes suffer from overtraining and overreaching. Thus, the trainers and athletes should ensure that their training plan is periodized along with slow progression.

Overtraining and overreaching can cause:
- Performance drop
- Weight loss and primary loss in muscle mass
- Chronic fatigue
- Elevated heart rate
- Elevated blood lactate levels during workout

If you are continuously feeling soreness in muscles, it's preferable to add a light workout day after 2-3 sessions for the same muscle group, which feeds fresh blood to the sore muscle groups, flushing waste products from the tissues.

Having contrast showers post-workout also removes metabolic waste and improves blood circulation in the body. Contrast shower demands submerging the body or parts into alternating bursts of cold and hot water for 1-2 minutes per burst. You might feel a mild discomfort, but repeat it for 5-6 times.

Cold water is a vasoconstrictor, and hot water is a vasodilator, hence the net effect of this improved circulation to the sore areas.

Reference - Page 100 : Quote from Tudor.O.Bompa
What is the Overtraining Syndrome? – IronMag Bodybuilding & Fitness Blog.
https://www.ironmagazine.com/2007/what-is-the-overtraining-syndrome/

Chapter 16: How to Measure Your Progress?

How do you measure your progress currently? Almost everyone who is a beginner checks their progress on a weighing scale. If your goal is fat loss and your weighing scale shows a dip, you feel you have made progress and vice versa if the goal is muscle gain.
That's not how our progress should be determined.

What if your goal is fat loss, but your weight is constant? It could be the case that you have gained muscle mass, which has improved your BMR, and you have lost some fat. That is decent progress!
The body composition scale is the best way to measure your progress. However, if you cannot afford to check on that, you will feel the difference in the fitting of your clothes. If you are losing inches and the weight is constant, you have lost fat and gained muscle mass.

Obviously, if you want to lose more fat mass than gain muscle mass, the ideal case would be to lose overall weight with more fat loss and some muscle gain. This will also happen with time if you are consistent. But let's talk about other ways to measure your progress, which a scale will not show, but you must count:
- Lifting more weight than before
- Having more energy throughout the day
- More stamina than before

- Improved form in the workouts
- Increased range of motion
- Increased reps or sets
- Better posture throughout the day
- No back pain
- More confidence
- More active mind at work
- Less binge eating and healthier food habits
- Lesser cravings

Or even doing one push-up when you were able to do none is progress that must not be neglected.

Chapter 17: Are Supplements Necessary?

Supplements are the concentrated form of nutrients that helps you fulfill your macronutrients or micronutrient requirements. They are not at all required if you can get all the needed macronutrients and micronutrients from natural sources in your diet.

When does a doctor recommend calcium, vitamin D or multivitamin tablets? When you are nutrition deficient, right? You reach that stage when you are not getting enough of that vitamin or mineral through your daily diet, and your body is unable to produce it.

So, if you realize that you are unable to complete your daily requirement of protein or any vitamin, is it really a bad idea to consume a supplement and avoid a stage where you need to visit a doctor for the same reason?

While some of the supplements are needed to meet the basic requirements, others are there to enhance athletic performance. The major question or fear related to supplements is the side effects of consuming those supplements, correct? Your fear is genuine because the name 'supplements' is a black box for a beginner.

Let's discuss some of the supplements that do not have side effects generally and, if consumed in adequate quantity, can enhance your performance.

Not consuming any one of them or taking one or more of them is your personal choice, but you should have knowledge about these supplements to stay away from myths. But your first rule should always be to get the maximum nutrition from natural sources and not try to replace them through supplements.

The major benefits of supplements are:
- It is a concentrated form of nutrition and very low in calories.
- Easily available in the market.
- It is beneficial to professional athletes and people who are involved in endurance and strength training and need a high amount of macros and micros.
- People with food allergies benefit from supplements as they contain digestive enzymes.

As a beginner, don't get overwhelmed by checking the list of supplements on the upcoming pages. You can just start with whey, and that too if you cannot fulfill your protein needs from daily meals. As you progress, get your blood tests done regularly to check the vitamin and mineral deficiency, and if required, you can add multivitamins.

Intermediate or advanced levels can decide wisely regarding other supplements if you really want to improve your athletic performance.

Disclaimer: All the supplements mentioned below do not have side effects on the general population unless you are allergic to some substance or have any medical condition. The recommended dosage mentioned depends on a lot of other factors, including the overall nutrition you are taking every day apart from consuming the supplement. So, please consume it only after consultation with your nutritionist and doctor.

Whey Protein

This is one of the most common supplements used to complete daily protein requirements. Whey protein is derived from the cheese-making process. When the protein of the milk is broken down, the liquid by-product of the milk is composed of 80% casein and 20% whey. This liquid whey is further pasteurized to be concentrated, and the final product is spray-dried into a powder form.

There are mainly three kinds of whey:

- Concentrate: It usually contains around 70-80% of proteins and is the most common and reasonable among all the three categories.
- Isolate: It usually contains around 85-90% proteins as it undergoes additional processing to minimize carbohydrates and fats, but the last process sometimes destroys the naturally occurring benefits of macronutrients and micronutrients. Isolate absorption is quicker than concentrated whey, and it is

recommended for lactose-intolerant people to concentrate.
- Hydrolysate or Hydrolyzed: It usually contains 90-94% proteins, and it is the ultra-pure form of whey. It is obtained through the pre-digestion process, and its absorption is the quickest. This is the costliest among all of them.

One scoop of whey protein is usually around 30g and around 120 Calories, and as per the category, it usually contains around 21-28g of protein and minimal carbohydrates or fats, even if it is concentrated whey.
It takes around 2 hours for whey to get absorbed completely, and hence, it is considered best when taken post-workout.

Whey protein usually contains decent levels of BCAA, and it is usually high in glutamine and arginine, along with essential and non-essential amino acids. Its benefit has been clinically proven in terms of increasing muscle growth and improving athletic performance. If your protein requirement for a day is 150g and you are struggling, it is fine to have one or two scoops of whey, but your major portion of proteins should come from food elements.

Recommended dosage: 1-2 scoops per day as training needs.

Casein Protein

Casein is also derived from milk, as explained above under the whey protein section, but they differ to a great extent, especially in terms of absorption. During the cheese-making process, enzymes are added to the milk, which causes casein in the milk to coagulate, separating it from the liquid whey.

In our body, proteins are broken into amino acids, which circulate in our bloodstream and finally get absorbed. Casein digestion is much slower than whey and hence is absorbed slower than whey.

It could take around 5-6 hours for one scoop of casein to get digested, and hence, the best time to consume casein is just before you go to sleep. Amino acids will be released in smaller amounts, and your muscles will not be protein-starved overnight, helping in muscle growth and recovery.

The most common casein in the market is micellar casein, which contains around 80% of protein by weight.

Casein increases the feeling of fullness and reduces appetite, and since almost all the lactose is removed during its manufacturing process, it is suitable for most lactose-intolerant people. But for people who are allergic to milk, you should avoid both casein and whey. Also, many casein products contain soy, so watch that if you are allergic to soy.

Casein contains around 26% less leucine (the most important BCAA) than whey.

Recommended dosage: 1-2 scoops per day as training needs.

Multivitamin & Multimineral
Multivitamins are available in the market in the form of tablets, which also contain all the essential multimineral. The quantity of vitamins and minerals differs slightly among different brands.

In general, it is recommended to have an annual health check-up, and in case you are deficient in vitamins or minerals, a doctor also suggests having a daily dosage of multivitamins.

If you are actively involved in physical activities, it is recommended that you ensure that you are not deficient in vitamins and minerals, so you can also include multivitamins in your routine after consulting with your doctor. If you are consuming them, make sure that you get your health check-up done regularly to know if you are not exceeding the upper limit of any vitamin or mineral since now we know that vitamins A, D, E and K are fat soluble and they could create toxicity if very high dosages are consumed for a prolonged time. However, most of the multivitamins have the vitamins and minerals in quantities less than or equal to RDA and even if you are getting those vitamins and minerals through natural sources, the probability of getting the dosage equivalent to what could create toxicity is quite low, but it is always good to be cautious

and get yourself tested to avoid any exceptional complications.
Most athletes are recommended to have multivitamins to avoid deficiency and to enhance performance.

Recommended dosage: 1 tablet per day or as directed by the physician.

Omega 3
Let's revisit the benefits of omega-3 – improving cardiovascular health, eye health and immune system. Also, they help in brain development, reducing inflammation, reducing fat in our liver and alleviating menstrual pain. We also discussed that omega-3 cannot be produced by our body, so we need to include them in our diet. In case we are unable to fulfil omega-3 requirements through natural sources of diet, there is no harm in taking omega-3 tablets.
Competitive athletes who consume between 2-4 grams of DHA and EPA have shown an increase in aerobic performance and strength.

Recommended dosage: 1 gram per day or as directed by the physician.

Creatine
Creatine is produced by our body and is also found in animal products. Cooking food items having creatine converts it into creatinine, which is excreted by our kidneys.

As of now, we know that during exercise, ATP is broken down by our cells to ADP (Adenosine Diphosphate), a phosphate molecule and energy.

ATP -> ADP + P (Energy released for cells)
ADP + P -> ATP (Energy absorbed from food)

Creatine, which is stored in muscle cells in the form of phosphocreatine, works as a source of immediate energy by aiding in the formation of new ATP (Adenosine Triphosphate).

Due to more ATP production, creatine indirectly helps in:
- Gaining muscle size
- Enhancing training intensity and power
- Increasing lean body mass
- Reducing lactate levels
- Reducing ammonia levels

Creatine retains water in your muscle cells, so you should consume a little more water (0.5-1L) if you are taking creatine supplements daily. Creatine monohydrate is the most common form of creatine, and a lot of studies have backed its effectiveness. Creatine monohydrate needs a loading phase followed by maintenance dosage. Below are two types of loading phases:

Quantity	Duration
15-20 grams per day	5-7 days
3-5 grams per day	Around 4 weeks

Athletes involved in explosive sports like powerlifting, boxing, football, hockey, sprinting, tennis, etc., are recommended to consume creatine supplements to improve performance.

Recommended dosage: 3-5 grams per day during maintenance phase (after loading).

Caffeine
Caffeine is commonly sold as an alertness aid drug. Almost every second person relies on caffeine to get the day started. It also offers other athletic benefits like:
- Decreases glycogen utilization
- Enhances physical performance
- Elevates fat oxidation
- Delays onset of fatigue
- Increases reaction time
- Helps in reducing water retention due to mild diuretic effect

Although caffeine increases physical and mental performance for a session, an overdose of caffeine and its related drugs could have side effects like:
- Insomnia and restlessness
- Faster heart beats
- Raises blood pressure
- Dehydration
- Digestive issues
- High intake may deplete calcium

High caffeine intake could also affect pregnant and lactating women in a negative way.

Comparatively, more water intake is required if you consume caffeine since it has a mild diuretic effect and causes frequent urination.

Caffeine is mainly found in coffee, tea, cola, chocolate sports drinks and pre-workout supplements.

Recommended dosage: Below 400mg daily is considered safe for non-pregnant adults, around 6 expresso shots of 30ml. Avoid exceeding 200mg of caffeine in a single dose.

Fats and slow metabolizer of caffeine
Suppose you are a fast metabolizer of caffeine. In that case, you can tolerate caffeine in comparatively larger amounts and experience more energy and alertness for a few hours after intake. In contrast, slow metabolizers of caffeine could be impacted by the stimulating effects of caffeine for a longer duration.
If you consume caffeine in the evening and face sleep issues at night, you are a slow metabolizer and avoid caffeine drinks in the second half of the day.

Ashwagandha
Ashwagandha is an Ayurvedic substance and is mainly known for its stress-relieving properties. It also has multiple benefits like:
- Aids in better sleep
- Enhanced athletic performance
- Improve concentration
- It may improve mental well-being

- It helps boost testosterone and increases men's fertility
- Reduces blood sugar levels
- It may improve brain health

Ashwagandha dosages may not be safe for pregnant and lactating women. Also, people with liver and thyroid problems or any other medication should consult a doctor before consumption. Some short-term effects may include vomiting, diarrhea or gastrointestinal issues.

Recommended dosage: It can vary depending on one's need, but less than 500mg is considered safe for the general population.

Gokhru

Gokhru, aka gokshura, aka Tribulus Terrestris, is another ayurvedic substance that is a small leafy plant sold in powder form in the market. It has several health benefits:
- Improving kidney functions
- Relieving urinary disorders
- Boosts testosterone and libido
- It may help lower blood sugar levels
- It helps in improving digestion
- Antioxidant properties that improve cardiac health

Although Gokhru has no significant side effects, it should be consumed in limited quantities, and in case it doesn't suit someone, you could face gastrointestinal issues.

Recommended dosage: 4-6 tsp if you prepare it using gokhru kwath. 100-250mg (1/2 to 1 tsp) can be taken from once to thrice a day as per requirement.

Citrulline Malate

Citrulline is a nitric oxide enhancer that converts into arginine (conditionally dispensable amino acid) and promotes nitrogen waste removal by removing ammonia from the blood, thereby relaxing blood vessels and improving blood flow. This results in:

- increasing muscle protein synthesis
- reduced muscle fatigue
- reduced soreness
- increases vascularity

Citrulline Malate is a combination of malic acid with citrulline, which helps to increase absorption rate and bioavailability. The bioavailability (i.e. the extent to which absorption occurs in the body) of L-arginine is relatively low (~20%), and hence citrulline malate is recommended to people who are into bodybuilding, heavy weightlifting or high-intensity training, so that they get an indirect advantage in competitions.

No potential side effects have been reported of citrulline on the general population when consumed under 10 grams per day. However, it can cause minor gastrointestinal problems in the short term in case it doesn't suit you as an exception. Pregnant and breastfeeding women should not consume it.

Recommended dosage: 3 to 6 grams per day can be taken in a divided dosage with not more than 3 grams in a single dosage.

Alanine & Beta-Alanine

Alanine is a dispensable amino acid that our body can produce. When glycogen stores are broken down into glucose, some of it is finally converted into alanine, which is transported to the liver through the bloodstream, and there it is again converted into glucose, thereby conserving energy through this cycle by maintaining glucose levels, which helps delay the onset of fatigue during the training.
It is beneficial to athletes who are into endurance training or weightlifting and who train for a longer duration.
Beta-alanine can increase the supply of carnosine. Carnosine has antioxidant properties, which are not only required for normal body functions but also improves training performance.

Recommended dosage: 3 to 5 grams per day can be taken in divided dosages, like consuming 1.5 grams twice per day.

Carnitine

Our body produces carnitine (L-carnitine), which transports the fatty acids into mitochondria for energy. It is beneficial to endurance professional athletes (like long-distance runners) who can see:

- Improvement in VO2 max
- Increased endurance
- Reduction in lactate levels
- Better anaerobic strength
- Preserve muscle glycogen and amino acids as energy sources during training
- Encourages the body to use more fat to be released for energy while training

Recommended dosage: Carnitine needs a loading of 2-4 grams daily around 2 weeks before the event to get performance-enhancing results. A single dosage should not be more than 2 grams at a time.

Ginseng

Ginseng has been researched for decades for improving athletic performance. Ginseng increases the body's oxygen supply due to the presence of germanium. It also contains antioxidants. Some of the significant benefits of ginseng include:

- Reduce lactic acid development while training
- Helps to improve VO2 max
- It may reduce inflammation due to antioxidant property
- Helps in enhancing motor skills coordination
- Improves brain function and mental performance
- Helps to boost immunity
- It may affect blood sugar levels

Some of the multivitamin/multimineral in the market have started adding ginseng to their tablets.

Recommended dosage: 100mg to 1g as per training needs.

I get a lot of questions about testosterone boosters and their consumption.
I would suggest a person get a blood test done to check the testosterone levels. If the levels are normal, you don't need to bother about the boosters. If the levels are low, you must always consult your doctor.

Personally, I consume whey, creatine monohydrate, multivitamins and omega-3, and I consume black coffee (caffeine) and a fruit (banana/apple) as a pre-workout. But, I started consuming all this after working out for over 12 years.

Chapter 18: Pre, Intra and Post-Workout Intake

Pre-workout, intra-workout and post-workout intake depend on one's goal and the kind of training they are involved in. Let's discuss it.

Pre-workout
If your meal is 30-60 minutes close to your workout, it is recommended that you consume simple carbohydrate (like banana or apple), which gets easily digested, and you get energy from them for your workout. You should avoid fats in pre-workout since they get digested slowly as compared to carbohydrates. Protein consumption before a workout can be in moderation.
However, if your meal is 2-3 hours before a workout, your meal can be balanced with the macronutrients.

Long training sessions: If you are going to train for a longer duration, like 2 hours or more, have some complex carbohydrates high in fiber, which are digested slowly. Also, include some proteins in your pre-workout.

Short training sessions: If you are not on an empty stomach (like you are training in the evening rather than early morning), you can go without pre-workout if your goal is fat loss. Remember that your glycogen stores might get depleted if your training session is stretched, and you will get energy from fatty acids. Keep yourself hydrated in order to avoid performance drops.

If you train in the morning hours and your intensity level could be high even if it is a short training session, it is recommended you don't train on an empty stomach since your body has already starved since night. You can have a fruit or any simple carbohydrate.

Caffeine (black coffee) can be used as a pre-workout to get some energy rush just before your training session.

Intra-workout
For low to moderate intensity levels in the morning hours, you can try to go on an empty stomach if you want to lose fat but keep an energy drink with you as intra-workout (a homemade energy drink could have water with a tbsp of glucose or electrolytes. Whey can be added as well as it has BCAA).
The need for electrolytes kicks in only if you are sweating too much to maintain water and salt balance. If you don't sweat much and you already had some pre-workout, you might not even feel the need for an intra-workout drink, which is absolutely fine.

If you are into professional endurance training for a longer duration or powerlifting, you must carry energy drinks with some electrolytes, simple carbohydrates and BCAA. Electrolytes will keep the salt and water balance. Simple carbohydrates will replenish your glycogen stores, and BCAA will ensure that leucine is replenished since if you are out of this amino acid, your protein synthesis for the day could be impacted.

Remember that you must sip the intra-workout drink gradually throughout the entire session and not gulp the entire drink at once.

Post-workout
You must include carbohydrates in your post-workout meal to replenish the glycogen stores along with some proteins. You can have Whey as a pre-workout, intra or post-workout. Ideally, the carbohydrates to proteins ratio in a workout meal should be 3:1, but in general, you can have a protein drink, a chicken breast, tofu (200g) soya chunks as a protein source along with oatmeal, veggies, salad, fruits, etc.

As a beginner, you must not worry about pre-, intra or post-workout much and focus on your daily macronutrient intake. As you progress in your training and feel the need as per your fatigue level, you can include the items gradually.

Chapter 19: Myths & Facts

Females should not lift heavy weights to avoid looking masculine.
A dominant hormone in females is estrogen, while in males, it is testosterone. Testosterone plays a vital role in muscle mass growth apart from other factors like sex drive, facial and pubic hair, etc. The average normal testosterone range for men is 300-1000 ng/dL, while it is 15-70 ng/dL for women. On average, women have around 20 times less testosterone than men, and hence, it requires much more effort for women to build that kind of muscle as compared to men.

Moreover, science also does not support the concept of different exercises for women and men. If you are scared because you have seen such exceptions where women have masculine physiques, it is highly likely that they might have taken testosterone separately to achieve that.

So, women – Please go ahead, lift weights and reap the benefits of weightlifting.

More cardio to lose fat.
More cardio to lose more muscles and metabolism. You lose overall weight, which includes water mass and muscle mass, and that degrades your metabolism when you do cardiovascular activities. Along with cardiovascular activities, you must do strength training to gain muscle mass, thereby increasing your metabolism, and hence, you

will burn more even in the resting state. Your nutrition part is the key, along with your workout, if your goal is to lose fat.

Do cardio after your strength training session since glycogen stores are depleted, and the body releases more energy from fatty acids.

My weight fluctuates a lot every day. I gained one pound in a day while I did nothing special since the last day.

Your weight fluctuation depends on the food and drinks you have consumed in the last 24-48 hours. The fluctuation you see in a day or even within a day is due to loss or gain in water weight, which is passed through urine, sweating, stool, etc.

Stop monitoring your weight every now and then. Check your body composition after a few weeks or a month to know the actual progress, and if you have gained some pounds but lost fat mass, you should be happy since you have gained muscle mass (if your water weight is almost constant). This fat loss is also seen in the loss of inches since one pound of muscle mass is lean and dense while one pound of fat mass is loose and flabby. So, gaining muscle and losing fat, even with constant weight, will make you look toned. Your clothes fitting speaks a lot about your progress even if you don't measure it on any scale.

Whey protein needs to be taken only when we workout.

Whey protein is not even needed if you workout and your daily protein requirements are being met with natural sources. Ultimately, everything comes up with daily requirements. Would you take vitamin D3 tablets if your D3 is too low and it is recommended by a doctor? In general, most people wait until it's too late and you need a doctor. It's always a great idea to understand the effects and side effects of anything rather than living in the darkness. If science has concluded that there are no side effects of consuming a substance, then it is the people who are talking about it, and that's a myth.

So, try to complete your daily requirement of protein through food items, but if you are struggling, there is no harm in consuming one or two scoops of whey protein. One scoop of whey protein generally contains 120 Calories and around 25g of proteins with traces of fat and carbs depending upon the brand and category of protein you are consuming.

Yes, the idea should always be to get more nutrition from natural sources rather than from supplements.

Add ample crunches to get rid of belly fat.
Do you think a person with a body fat of 25% can have six-pack abs if the person does 500 crunches per day? Understand the fact that spot reduction is not possible. Body fat is reduced proportionally from your entire body, and crunches will help you strengthen your core muscles but won't remove belly fat. Following a macronutrient-balanced diet as per your goal, along with strength and cardiovascular training, is the way to reduce overall fat. Follow

the process with consistency and discipline, and you will achieve such results as a byproduct with time.

Too much soy increases estrogen levels, decreases testosterone levels, and men can get male boobs.
We must have heard this a lot. Soy does have phytoestrogens, which have properties similar to estrogen. Estrogen helps in reproductive and bone health for male physiology, and the amount of soy you can practically consume in a day, even if you consume it daily, will not increase your estrogen levels to such an extent that a man can get male boobs. Also, soy does not decrease testosterone. Soy is a great source of proteins, carbohydrates and unsaturated fats. Moreover, boiling or cooking soya chunks decreases the phytoestrogen content, which is another good news for you. Feel free to include it in your daily meal if you like it.

We should not consume more than 30 grams of protein in a meal since the body won't be able to absorb it.
The excess protein you consume in a meal is stored in the amino acids pool in the intestine and is provided to the body when required. However, if you are consistently talking about a higher amount of proteins and your body is unable to utilize it in the form of energy, the excess proteins get converted into fat through the process of gluconeogenesis.
Imagine a 120 kg wrestler consuming 300 grams of proteins and taking ten meals with 30

grams of proteins per meal with the fear of getting extra proteins removed through waste from the body. We need to figure out how much protein we can digest and increase it gradually from our current limit accordingly if needed.

Drink jeera water, lime water, apple cider vinegar or other liquid to get rid of body fat.
Drinking or eating any liquid or food item will not help you lose fat. Every item has zero to some calories, which adds up to your calorie budget. Also, the food or beverage you consume goes into your stomach and bloodstream. There is no interaction of any food item directly with the adipose tissue, which can help in fat loss. Yes, replacing a morning beverage of 150 Calories with almost zero calories liquid would indirectly help in overall daily calorie intake, provided other food items are constant. Ultimately, a calorie deficit diet along with physical activity will only help you to lose fat.

More short meals in a day increases metabolism.
Whether you consume 2-3 meals or 5-6 meals, if your overall calorie intake of the day is the same in both cases, it will not affect your metabolism, absorption, or any other factor. Yes, if your daily calorie budget is 2,500 Calories, it could be difficult to consume it in 2 meals, but if you are able to consume it without any gastrointestinal issues, it doesn't make any difference to your metabolism. You can have a meal when you feel hungry, or you can train your mind as per your routine and availability

to have 2-3 or 4-5 meals without worrying about other factors.

Is Intermittent Fasting (IF) safe to achieve results?

Yes, intermittent fasting has several benefits. It demands consuming food in a window of 8:16 (8 hours of eating against 16 hours of not eating). Hence, the window causes people to eat a comparatively lesser number of meals, which helps in the reduction of blood sugar levels, making it hard for cancer cells to grow since cancer cells feed on glucose. The IF also reduces oxidative stress inflammation in the body and improves other metabolic features, which is good for brain health.

While performing IF, the only thing you need to take care of is your calorie budget and macronutrient ratio as per your goal. With the idea of taking a lesser number of meals, people start consuming less and stay nutrition deprived, through which they definitely lose weight but in an unhealthy way by compromising muscle mass, metabolism and other hormonal functions.

Ghee is good for health, and you should have it plentiful.

Cow ghee has nutrients like vitamins A, E, and K, omega-3 fatty acids, and conjugated linolenic acid, but also remember that ghee has 99.8% saturated fat, which means one tablespoon of ghee has around 15g grams of fat. Considering your daily macronutrients limit and unsaturated fats consumption, you can include some ghee in your diet. It is also absolutely fine to avoid it since there is no special nutrient that is only available in ghee and no other item.

Collagen supplements are good for the skin to achieve anti-ageing effects.

The bioavailability of collagen supplements is quite low (20-25%), which means it gets absorbed poorly. Our focus should be to work on the factors that could impair collagen production. Alcohol, smoking, sedentary and unhealthy lifestyles are the major factors that impair its production. Also, there is insufficient research that supports the benefits of oral consumption of collagen. So, instead of running after collagen supplements, work on the root cause to enhance collagen production.

The more sweating during a workout, the more calories are burned.

Through the thermoregulation process, our body regulates temperature through sweat in order to return to the core temperature when the temperature of our body is increased through heat. More sweating has nothing to do with the burning of the fat. If that had been the case, people would have been sitting all day switching off fans and ACs to lose fat. Feel free to workout in AC, and too much heat and sweating also impairs your performance by losing water and electrolytes.

Consuming rice or carbohydrates in the night makes you fat.
The major calories of rice come from carbohydrates. Unless and until your daily macronutrients are balanced, it hardly matters if you are consuming rice daily, avoiding it completely, or having it in your first or last meal. Rice or carbohydrates don't make you fat!

Chapter 20: Closure

Thank you for staying till the end of this book. There are still many more things that I could have told you with regard to training, but the idea of this book was to share the basic trusted process that has been followed by people whose life has been transformed.
I see a lot of people involved in physical activities or going to the gym, but they fail to understand where exactly they are failing. In order to cherish your favourite meals for a lifetime, you must understand the basics of fitness and nutrition to apply them.

You might hear people coming up with different theories and science in the fitness industry, and the research is a continuous process, so you will continue to hear them throughout your life. Your focus should not be to dive into the ocean of theories. It would help if you started with a swimming pool where you can learn the basics to add fitness to your lifestyle and routine. You need to figure out what works best for you as per your goal, but what has been mentioned in this book are the basics that would work for everyone unless you already have some medical condition where you need to consult your doctor!

Doors of fitness trainers and sports nutritionists come before the doors of doctors if you do not have a medical condition. However, if you have already reached a medical condition, you first need a doctor and then a fitness trainer because you are late in the game. Although better late than never, you should still start your fitness journey with a doctor's consultation.

Please stop blaming situations and other external factors for your health. Yes, there would be factors that you couldn't have avoided, but now is the time to find time for yourself and make things better. No matter how close your family or friends are to you, you are the one who has to go through the pain if your health goes down. Others can empathize with you, but no one can gift you an active lifestyle. Even the richest person can buy all the tools and equipment, but ultimately, the person will have to workout and maintain a balanced diet to earn a healthy and active lifestyle.

The all-in or all-out approach doesn't work in fitness! You might not feel the same energy level on all the days, but just keep going even if the efforts are not 100% every day; just show up!

So, all the best for your fitness journey!
My upcoming book of this course will cover the knowledge about nutrition and will uncover the secrets to cheating wisely at social gatherings, understanding label readings and choosing items for your diet as per your plan and routine.

Did this book help you in some way? If so, I would really appreciate your honest review so that it would help other people find the right book for their needs. This will also give me motivation to write more content and share more knowledge that I have.

You can scan the below QR code to leave a review!

Thank you for taking the time to share the review!

Printed in Great Britain
by Amazon